THIRD EDITION

PROJECT PLANNING
AND MANAGEMENT

A Guide for Nurses and
Interprofessional Teams

Edited by

JAMES L. HARRIS, PHD, MBA, APRN-BC, CNL, FAAN
Professor of Nursing
University of South Alabama
Mobile, Alabama

LINDA ROUSSEL, PHD, RN, NEA-BC, CNL, FAAN
Visiting Professor
Texas Woman's University
Denton, Texas

CATHERINE DEARMAN, PHD, RN
Educational Consultant
President and CEO
D&D Consulting
Mobile, Alabama

PATRICIA L. THOMAS, PHD, MSN, RN, NEA-BC, ACNS-BC, CNL, FACHE, FNAP
Assistant Dean for Practice and Associate Professor
Cook DeVos Health Science Center
Kirkhof College of Nursing
Grand Valley State University
Grand Rapids, Michigan

JONES & BARTLETT
LEARNING

World Headquarters
Jones & Bartlett Learning
5 Wall Street
Burlington, MA 01803
978-443-5000
info@jblearning.com
www.jblearning.com

Jones & Bartlett Learning books and products are available through most bookstores and online booksellers. To contact Jones & Bartlett Learning directly, call 800-832-0034, fax 978-443-8000, or visit our website, www.jblearning.com.

Substantial discounts on bulk quantities of Jones & Bartlett Learning publications are available to corporations, professional associations, and other qualified organizations. For details and specific discount information, contact the special sales department at Jones & Bartlett Learning via the above contact information or send an email to specialsales@jblearning.com.

Production Credits

VP, Product Management: David D. Cella
Director of Product Management: Amanda Martin
Product Manager: Rebecca Stephenson
Product Assistant: Anna-Maria Forger
Production Manager: Carolyn Rogers Pershouse
VMO Manager: Sara Kelly
Vendor Manager: Juna Abrams
Senior Marketing Manager: Jennifer Scherzay
Product Fulfillment Manager: Wendy Kilborn
Composition: S4Carlisle Publishing Services
Project Management: S4Carlisle Publishing Services
Cover Design: Kristin E. Parker
Text Design: Kristin E. Parker
Director of Rights & Media: Joanna Gallant
Rights & Media Specialist: Wes DeShano
Rights & Media Specialist: John Rusk
Media Development Editor: Shannon Sheehan
Cover Image (Title Page, Chapter Opener): ©Shuoshu/ DigitalVision Vectors/Getty Images
Printing and Binding: Sheridan Books, Inc.
Cover Printing: Sheridan Books, Inc.

Library of Congress Cataloging-in-Publication Data
Names: Harris, James L. (James Leonard), 1956- editor. | Roussel, Linda, editor. | Thomas, Patricia L., 1961- editor. | Dearman, Catherine, editor.
Title: Project planning and management : a guide for nurses and interprofessional teams / [edited by] James Harris, Linda A. Roussel, Patricia (Tricia) Thomas, Catherine Dearman.
Other titles: Project planning and management (Harris)
Description: Third edition. | Burlington, Massachusetts : Jones & Bartlett Learning, [2020] | Includes bibliographical references and index.
Identifiers: LCCN 2018007520 | ISBN 9781284147056 (paperback)
Subjects: | MESH: Nursing--organization & administration | Clinical Nursing Research--methods | Program Development--methods | Planning Techniques | Interprofessional Relations
Classification: LCC RT89 | NLM WY 105 | DDC 610.73068--dc23 LC record available at https://lccn.loc.gov/2018007520

6048

Printed in the United States of America
22 21 20 19 18   10 9 8 7 6 5 4 3 2 1

Contents

Chapter 5 Literature Synthesis and Organizational Alignment to Project Interventions and Implementation 75

Catherine Dearman, Lolita Chappel-Aiken, and Katrina Davis

Chapter 6 The Institutional Review Board Process 85

Catherine Dearman, Dionne Roberts, and Lolita Chappel-Aiken

Chapter 7 Synergistic Interprofessional Teams: Essential Drivers of Person-Centered Care 103

Patricia L. Thomas and Janet E. Winter

Chapter 8 Managing the Interprofessional Project Team 121

James L. Harris and Kathryn M. Ward-Presson

Chapter 9 Making the Case for a Project: Needs Assessment 137

Carolyn Thomas Jones and Linda Roussel

Chapter 10 Using Findings from the Clinical Needs Assessment to Develop, Implement, and Manage Sustainable Projects. 157

Linda Roussel, Shea Polancich, and Murielle S. Beene

Chapter 11 Role of Information Technology in Project Planning and Management. 177

James L. Harris and Todd Harlan

Chapter 12 Developing Metrics That Support Project Plans, Interventions, and Programs 193

Patricia L. Thomas

**Chapter 13 Measuring the Value
 of Projects Within
 Organizations,
 Healthcare
 Systems,
 and Globally. 221**

Patricia L. Thomas and Michael Bleich

**Chapter 14 Disseminating
 Results of
 Meaningful Projects
 and Their
 Management. 233**

*Catherine Dearman and
 Lolita Chappel-Aiken*

Preface

The primary function of a textbook is to be a reference for students, faculty, teams, and consumers of care. Healthcare organizations are challenged to maintain a competitive edge. What one views as a crisis situation in a healthcare organization, the crisis generates creativity in another. Meaningful interprofessional quality projects must add value, contribute to evidence, What one views as a crisis situation in a healthcare organization, generates creativity in another, and provide sustainable outcomes for survival in today's healthcare market. Our dedication as educators, administrators, clinicians, and nurse researchers led us to update the second edition of the text to meet the constant change and activities within organizations. As healthcare environments continue to require up-to-date information and evidence-based innovative practices, interprofessional project teams and learning collaboratives have formed. The collective talents and insights of these teams and collaboratives are necessary in order to meet the challenges of providing quality, safe, and efficient care in a turbulent environment. As interprofessional teams work together, new behaviors develop and an understanding of the contributions from other disciplines emerges.

We contend that the content in the *Third Edition* is not all-inclusive but, rather provides a snapshot for designing, updating, and evaluating interprofessional quality improvement projects that transcend across the continuum of care. This edition's content provides a foundation for successful project planning and management, interprofessional team management, implementation science, team synergy, and use of needs assessments to shape projects. Based on comments from students, faculty, biomedical librarians, and institutional review boards, we added material on influences and determinants of projects, team science, and literature synthesis and organizational alignments to projects in this edition.

We hope that the information provided in the *Third Edition* will encourage interprofessional teams to join forces and develop projects that change healthcare delivery. A team's vision serves as a compass to guide meaningful projects and spread evidence that adds value and engenders sustainable change.

James L. Harris
Linda Roussel
Catherine Dearman
Patricia L. Thomas

Acknowledgments

My colleagues and I acknowledge each of the contributors of this text, mentors who have guided our careers, and the review comments from various individuals and disciplines represented. In an era of constant changes in society and health care, the call for action by transformational leaders who support and encourage interprofessional quality improvement team activities is paramount if organizations are to survive. Projects create pathways for patient-centered care, opportunities for synergy, evidence-based knowledge creation and spread, and directions for meeting the Triple and Quadruple Aims.

To our families and colleagues who supported this edition, we offer our thanks for the encouragement and guidance. To the staff at Jones & Bartlett Learning, your consistent support and unwavering direction are equally appreciated.

James L. Harris
Linda Roussel
Catherine Dearman
Patricia L. Thomas

Contributors

Murielle S. Beene, DNP, MBA, MPH, MS, RN-BC, PMP, FAAN
Chief Nursing Informatics Officer
Department of Veterans Affairs
Washington, DC

Michael Bleich, PhD, RN, NEA-BC, FNAP, FAAN
President and CEO
NursDynamics
Ballwin, MO

Lolita Chappel-Aiken, PhD, RN
Chair of Graduate Programs
Division of Nursing
School of Health Sciences
Winston-Salem State University
Winston-Salem, NC

Clista Clanton, MSLS
Biomedical Library
University of South Alabama
Mobile, AL

Katrina Davis, DNP(c), RN
Division of Nursing
School of Health Sciences
Winston-Salem State University
Winston-Salem, NC

Catherine Dearman, PhD, RN
Educational Consultant
President and CEO
D&D Consulting
Mobile, AL

Todd Harlan, DNP, RN
Associate Professor of Nursing
Chair, Community Mental Health
  Nursing
University of South Alabama
Mobile, AL

James L. Harris, PhD, MBA, APRN-BC, CNL, FAAN
Professor of Nursing
University of South Alabama
Mobile, AL

Carolyn Thomas Jones, DNP, MSPH, RN
Lead Instructor, Master of Applied
  Clinical and Preclinical
  Research
Assistant Professor of Nursing,
  College of Nursing
The Ohio State University
Columbus, OH

Shea Polancich, PhD, RN
Assistant Professor of Nursing
University of Alabama, Birmingham
Birmingham, AL

Bettina Riley, PhD, RN
Associate Professor Nursing
University of South Alabama
Mobile, AL

Dionne Roberts, PhD, FNP-C, CNE
Associate Professor & FNP/DNP
  Program Director
FNP (MSN and DNP) Director
Winston-Salem State University
Winston-Salem, NC

Linda Roussel, PhD, RN, NEA-BC, CNL, FAAN
Visiting Professor
Texas Woman's University
Denton, TX

Patricia L. Thomas, PhD, MSN, RN, NEA-BC, ACNS-BC, CNL, FACHE, FNAP
Assistant Dean for Practice and
  Associate Professor
Cook DeVos Health Science Center
Kirkhof College of Nursing
Grand Valley State University
Grand Rapids, MI

Janet E. Winter, DNP, MPA, RN
Associate Dean of Undergraduate
  Programs in Nursing
Cook DeVos Health Science Center
Kirkhof College of Nursing
Grand Valley State University
Grand Rapids, MI

CASE STUDY CONTRIBUTORS

Jennifer Anne Blalock, RN
Graduate Student
University of South Alabama
Mobile, AL

Amy Campbell, DNP, MSN, RN
Assistant Professor
University of South Alabama
Mobile, AL

Wes Garrison, DNP, RN, MBA
Associate Chief Nursing Officer
Northeast Georgia Medical Center
Gainesville, GA

Theodora Ledford, MSN, RN, CNL
Clinical Nurse Leader
Charles George VA Medical Center
Asheville, NC

Jacqueline M. Lollar, DNP, RN
Assistant Professor of Nursing
University of South Alabama
Mobile, AL

K. Michele Lyons, MN, RN
Southeastern Louisiana University
Hammond, LA

Margaret Mitchell, DNP, MN, FNP
Former Graduate Student
University of South Alabama
Mobile, AL

Terri Poe, DNP, RN, NE-BC
Chief Nursing Officer
University of Alabama Hospitals
Birmingham, AL

Heather Surcouf, DNP, MSN, BSN, FNP
Methodist Health Systems Foundation
Slidell, LA

Kathryn M. Ward-Presson, DNP, RN, NEA-BC
Ward Consulting Partners, LLC
Jonas Scholar in Veterans Healthcare
  Alumni
Raleigh, NC

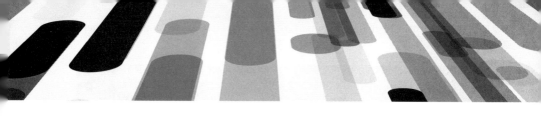

CHAPTER 1

Key Foundations of Successful Project Planning and Management

James L. Harris

CHAPTER OBJECTIVES

1. Differentiate between a project, a plan, and their management.
2. Prioritize needs to support a project plan and program plan, program sustainability, and an operating budget.
3. Combine the components of project planning to design a value-based program.
4. Identify requisite skills and tools for the development, initiation, evaluation, and dissemination of quality improvement projects and their continuous management.
5. Generate processes necessary to manage individuals and system-wide projects and teams in virtual environments.

KEY TERMS

Continuous quality improvement
Management
Project budget
Project management
Project plan
Return on investment

Stakeholders
Sustainability
Teams
Value
Virtual environment

ROLES

Communicator	Leader
Designer	Manager
Educator	

PROFESSIONAL VALUES

Integrity	Patient-centeredness

CORE COMPETENCIES

Analysis	Evidence-based practice
Appreciative inquiry	Integration
Assessment	Leadership
Communication	Risk anticipation and mitigation
Critical thinking	Systems thinking
Emotional intelligence	

▶ Introduction

Regardless of the industry, transformation is central to the future success of a global economy. What was once merely pondered by many in the healthcare arena has now evolved into sustainable project plans and value-based programs that are driven by the basic instinct of survival. New vistas of appreciative inquiry await a mindful revolution of individuals and global leaders dedicated to seamless integration and coordination of projects that will ultimately benefit the health and economic well-being of society (Robert Wood Johnson Foundation, 2014). Appreciative inquiry provides a framework for strategic project planning highlighting current industry trends and is a catalyst for organizational change (Stratton-Berkessel, 2010).

As individuals consider the daunting task of improving health and well-being at the microlevel of a global society, they must recognize that having a project idea and actually implementing it are two different things. Understanding the scope of a project, the stakeholder involvement, team dynamics, economics, the political environment, and the actual requirements can lead many to become daunted and enter a state of paralysis. In the healthcare industry, the path to an innovative project that will add **value** from the microlevel and potential globally centers around six elements as identified by the World Health Organization (WHO, 2008):

1. Addressing the service to be delivered
2. Financing
3. Governance
4. Workforce
5. Information systems
6. Supply management

Successful planning and implementation of any project are supported by the notion that effective system strengthening requires systems thinking and attention to how the parts work together to create a seamless whole (Crisp, 2010). As knowledge is gained from project outcomes, knowledge transfer becomes an imperative. Evidence is spread and systems of care are strengthened and sustained. This is relevant in the current environment, where the focus of work is on obtaining the right outcomes, as opposed to past decades, where performing the right processes was emphasized (Porter-O'Grady & Malloch, 2015). Equally, the relevance is increasingly predominant in a market driven by value-based versus volume-based care delivery and reimbursement (Frist, 2016).

This chapter focuses on differences in a project, the project plan, the project budget, the project's **management**, and strategies used to prioritize project needs. Linking value to the project design, requisite skills, and tools necessary for a successful and sustainable project are then described. As work environments continue to become more virtual, managing project **teams** remotely also becomes a concern; such virtual management is discussed in this chapter.

▶ Projects, Project Plans, and Project Management Defined

The genesis of any project is planning, but ongoing management of the project is essential as well. All projects have a beginning, duration, and an end, which collectively constitute the project's life cycle. Project outcomes may be, for example, adopted in the form of evidence-based guidelines or seen as opportunities to conduct additional inquiry and validation studies prior to including them in practice. It is critical, however, not to immediately adopt findings from a small project, as they may not be generalizable to a broader context. According to Peters (1999), approximately 50% of the work completed in organizations may be considered as projects. Many staff working on projects as de facto members or managers may not possess the critical path and earned value analysis skills, which are key to orchestrating and managing a project from inception to completion (Lewis, 2011).

What is a project? According to the Project Management Institute (2013), a project is a temporary endeavor focused on producing a unique operational entity (e.g., a product, a service, or a result differing from that obtained in prior projects). Juran (1992) describes a project as a problem scheduled for solution. While the word "problem" may elicit a negative emotion, it does not necessarily imply negativity. Outcomes can create a positive problem, such as a new product or clinical procedure directed at reducing urinary tract infections among elderly individuals or addressing other clinical phenomena. In any event, the project should be based on the notion of accomplishing a goal for systems, **stakeholders**, and/or customers.

When does the project begin? A series of activities and actions precedes the initiation of a project. One fundamental consideration is readying the project environment by identifying and validating the need for the project, developing the plan, and obtaining system buy-in and/or approval from stakeholders.

A **project plan** encompasses several components that collectively culminate in a realistic and well-planned sequence of actions and processes. The project plan goes beyond a general project scope and includes the details necessary to make a meaningful and value-based addition to a work unit or an entire system. According to Tuthill (2014), the project plan includes a budget, a work and activity breakdown and schedule, an overall project schedule, and any supporting documents. Haughey (2014) identified other, related parts of the project plan, including project goals, deliverables, schedule, and supporting documents (human resources, communications, and risk management plans). Additionally, other project plan considerations were outlined by Billows (2014), whose project plan template provides for scope definition, major deliverables, risk identification, team resource requirements, and decomposing individual tasks. A variety of project-planning programs are available commercially and often used by larger, more complex projects within systems.

Thinking and rethinking what one needs or desires in relation to the project plan are key aspects of planning captured by Merrifield (2009). This author identified three important "rethinking questions" for any student or project planning team:

1. Does the project exactly correlate with any of the organization's key business goals?
2. Does the project have a strong connection to the organization's brand or corporate identity?
3. Does the effort required for the project result in increased organizational performance and change the value of the project to achieve organizational effectiveness?

What is **project management**? The *Project Management Body of Knowledge (PMBOK) Guide* defines project management as "application of knowledge, skills, tools, and techniques to project activities to meet project requirements. Project management is accomplished through the application and integration of the project management processes of initiating, planning, executing, monitoring and controlling, and closing" (Project Management Institute, 2013, p. 6). Of interest, the *PMBOK Guide* has, as its primary objective, the explanation of how each of the processes may be accomplished in practice.

While consistent management of activities is essential for project completion, project management extends beyond managing and scheduling activities. Project management entails a combination of tools, people, and systems (Lewis, 2011). Tools may include computers, software packages, and daily planners. People include organizations and project teams who engage in processes geared toward goal accomplishment within systems. Management of people may present as a challenge in this endeavor, and leaders and communicators must use multiple skills to coach and mentor individuals toward achieving the common goal. The manager's emotional intelligence may be tested along the way, as will be discussed further in this chapter.

Regardless of the depth or breadth of the project, plan, and management, the various stages of the project life cycle must not be neglected. Tuthill (2014) identified this cycle as having four phases:

1. Initiating the project (including identifying customer-driven factors and obtaining leadership approval and support)
2. Planning (including human and physical resources)
3. Executive (monitors, control, and cycle of efforts)
4. Project closure (training, operations, and support)

Project planning across the life cycle should also take into account the project's feasibility, value, key drivers for success, skills and tools needed, and processes whereby project teams may be managed in **virtual environments**. Virtual work environments have gained popularity in the last decade as more employees work from distant locations. Virtual work environments are advantageous for a company as fewer expenditures are dedicated for office space, supplies, and indirect costs (Bloch, 2017).

▶ Prioritizing Needs That Support Project Plans and Programs

The challenges facing the healthcare industry today are complicated by rising expenditures, quality and safety concerns, changes in service needs and expectations, new technologies, provider shortages, and care reform legislation, to name a few of the myriad influences in this environment. In such a complex and rapidly changing landscape, identifying what needs to be done and determining how to quickly accomplish a task is essential if projects are supported, sustained, and manageable and if they are to truly impact organizations and programs. To ensure effectiveness of a project, one must start by prioritizing the primary need and any evidentiary basis that underpins a need for change and rapid response. Otherwise, the feasibility of any project will be jeopardized from its inception.

Which steps should a student or project team take to prioritize needs? An assessment of the environment is an initial step, which is then followed by development of a strategy. Strategy planning must include consideration of any unintended consequences of the project. This requires the identification of "what if" scenarios and solutions with projected and/or desired measurable outcomes.

Assessing the Environment

New circumstances require a "new state" that is not known and must emerge from development of a vision, innovation, and learning. Such an effort requires a fundamental shift in mindset, organizing principles, behavior, culture, and infrastructure. A critical mass within the organization or work unit must operate from a new mindset and behavior if change is to be achieved.

A prudent individual who is beginning to develop a project plan must also be aware of the constancy of change. Change is not necessarily a linear or sequential process but rather may appear at any point during an environmental assessment. Scholars have gleaned much from studies of complex adaptive systems in relation to change. Specifically, change cannot be specified and managed in detail. Small changes in critical elements or leverage points, however, have the potential to engender large changes. Leadership, values, and culture are important for achieving any change, whether that change is implemented by a student engaging in a capstone project or through a system-wide initiative (Plsek & Greenhalgh, 2001). Change can have a profound impact on developing the best strategy necessary to initiate and complete a project. Being attuned to emerging conditions, forces, and trends may provide an individual with insight into the convergence of subtleties that create and affect work environments and the readiness for change (Porter-O'Grady & Malloch, 2015).

When assessing the environment, two fundamental activities should occur sequentially: an assessment of strengths, weaknesses, opportunities, and threats (SWOT analysis) and a gap analysis. Input from both the SWOT analysis and the gap analysis are used in all systems. Output from one type of analysis can be used as input for the other, and vice versa. In completing the SWOT analysis, all levels (micro, meso, and macro) must be examined, as information from each area can provide valuable insights when delimiting the scope of the project and strategies to control positive and negative factors affecting success.

Closely linked to the SWOT analysis is the gap analysis, in which individuals seek to establish the root problem and collect evidence that supports the need for engaging in the project. A gap analysis compares actual performance with potential performance, such as that demonstrated via performance measures. This type of analysis may also be referred to as a needs assessment. During the gap analysis, the current state of the system, factors needed to reach a target or benchmark, and a plan to fill the gap may be identified. This type of assessment is very beneficial in all systems, but especially in today's healthcare arena, where the impetus is on identifying areas with performance deficits that impact resource allocation, planning, productivity, and quality indicators.

Both SWOT analysis and gap analysis are useful to a system, and their findings can be drilled down to identify a common denominator. Indeed, both types of analyses can be used in different contexts with different meanings. **TABLE 1-1** describes the different uses of each from a healthcare perspective.

Strategy Development

Upon completion and analysis of the SWOT and gap analysis, the strategy is selected and developed to address the priority need(s). As noted by Lewis (2011), strategy is the overall approach to a problem. Strategy is very important because it is often possible to generate multiple alternative solutions to a problem. It is not uncommon for students to take away differing ideas from assessment data and then find themselves conflicted about which problem to tackle first. Should the problem selected be of personal interest, rather than based on system needs? This type of question is why strategy is so important.

In the situation where several problems are identified (based on personal preference and system need), one technique is to rank order them by engaging a team for their prioritization. Engaging others in the process engenders buy-in and ownership of a

TABLE 1-1 SWOT and Gap Analysis: Uses in Health Care

SWOT Analysis	Gap Analysis
Hospital comparison data	Patient discharge by 11 a.m.
Eliminate hospital-acquired pressure ulcers (Zero HAP Program)	Reduce emergency department wait times by: 15% in Quarter 1 75% in Quarters 2–4 90% for fiscal year
Build comprehensive cardiac care center	Streamline waits for elective cardiac studies

successful project. Consideration should be given to the environmental assessment, various variables, and data points available in this process.

The selected strategy should also address various levels of need—micro-, meso-, and macrosystem needs—depending on the scope of the project. Many healthcare systems today maintain a list of quality improvement projects at a variety of levels needing intervention, as suggested by root-cause analysis findings, internal focused reviews, and/or external reviews. Regardless of whether a "wish list" of projects is provided, any student engaged in a capstone project should complete the environmental assessment and strategy development steps. This creates opportunities for gleaning new information and learning more about the process—knowledge that will prove useful when the student is engaged in or leading projects.

As previously stated, anticipating unintended consequences and managing them to achieve measurable and desired outcomes are steps that cannot be ignored. Unanticipated and unintended consequences are present in all environments. Many such consequences can be traced to prior decisions and attempts to solve problems without projecting those actions' long-range consequences or providing for risk mitigation. It is human nature to want to do the right thing. Without careful analysis of issues and engagement of stakeholders, however, situations may occur that have deleterious effects. Risk anticipation and mitigation are therefore needed, as is identification of ways to avoid and overcome problems while preserving the intent and integrity of the project.

Good communication at all levels is a cornerstone of successful projects. Consensus on a final project that is clearly presented and mutually agreed upon is needed before the project starts. Many individuals and project teams present a succinct project plan or business case in a concise format. Gaining the support of team members and all stakeholders early on in the process becomes essential to the ongoing sustainability of the project, as, ultimately, programs depend on both individual and collective input. Milestones must be detailed and met, although these points may be communicated in different ways.

▶ The Project Budget

A well-developed **project budget** is based on objectives and a detailed estimate of all costs required from inception to completion. Project budgets should be flexible, have standards, and use available sources first to avoid unnecessary costs. A typical project budget includes costs for staff labor, materials and their procurement, ongoing operation costs, other direct costs such as travel and education, and indirect costs that support the project such as building expenses. The proposed budget provides information to develop a cost-benefit analysis and a **return on investment** expressed in a ratio as net profit divided by total investment times 100 (Finkler, Jones, & Kovner, 2013).

Harrin (2015) identified four sequential steps to a well-planned project budget. First, break down the tasks. Breaking down the work and listing what is needed for the project's completion is important from the onset. Second, estimate the tasks based on expert knowledge and past experiences. Third, total the estimates in order to create the total for the planned budget. Fourth, add in any extras that may arise unexpectedly as the project proceeds. A 10% contingency is common in case the costs were poorly estimated. An example of a project budget template is provided in **TABLE 1-2**.

TABLE 1-2 Project Budget Template				
Line Item		**FY 07–08**		
	Labor	**Material**	**Other**	**FY Total**
Total				

Total Project Budget: $_____   **Return on Investment:** _____%

▶ Value-Based Project Attributes for Project Sustainment and Management

The healthcare system in the United States remains the costliest of all developed countries, with healthcare expenditures expected to increase from 17% to 20% of the gross domestic product by 2020 (Centers for Medicare and Medicaid Services, 2010). Regardless of the country, however, all health systems are challenged to create greater value from the resources dedicated to health care (Institute for Healthcare Improvement [IHI], 2014). Porter-O'Grady and Malloch (2015) contend that clinical work processes today must derive value from a purpose directed toward a desired outcome and emphasize work that achieves real value, rather than focusing on the work itself. Achieving high value for patients must be the primary goal for any project. If value improves, all stakeholders can benefit, and the economic sustainability of programs and the healthcare system will, in turn, increase (Porter, 2010).

Since value is expressed relative to costs, efficiency and accountability should be shared among all individuals involved. This reinforces the need to involve others in any project, concentrating on integrated activities where all stakeholders are accountable for value-based outcomes (Porter, 2010). Projects planned with the IHI Triple Aim (IHI, 2014) and Quadruple Aim (Bodenheimer & Sinsky, 2014) in mind can optimize health system performance, improve the work life of healthcare providers, and engage other stakeholders. But why consider the Triple and Quadruple Aims when planning projects? The dimensions of the Triple Aim—namely, improving the patient's experience of care, improving population health, and reducing the per-capita cost of care—are foundational to harnessing a broad range of community determinants of health and services, where others are engaged and a seamless journey of care follows.

As projects are planned and all components are considered, adopting a strategy that will achieve the Triple and Quadruple Aims can be realized as solutions to problems are identified further upstream, beyond the inpatient setting. Fundamentally, the value proposition of the project, thought of mathematically as "Value = Quality/Cost," extends beyond a unit or acute care setting to community-based care (Lighter, 2011). Ideally, the burden of illness is decreased through coordinated care, and the per-capita costs are stabilized or reduced.

Well-designed projects with measurable outcomes solidify evidence-based practice and support further inquiry. One means to project value that is commonly used by organizations, accrediting and certification agencies, and students is the six industry services characteristics highlighted by the Institute of Medicine (IOM):

1. Safe
2. Effective
3. Patient-centered
4. Timely
5. Efficient
6. Equitable (IOM, 2001; Steinwachs & Hughes, 2008)

Regardless of how small or large the project is, all well-developed and well-executed projects are driven by key markers of value and success. These key markers include innovation, inclusiveness, an evidence-based foundation, and transparency. New innovative practices and technology are spurred daily by individual and group brainstorming, which often serves as the originating point for value-driven projects that sustain effective programs. Including others in any project idea and design can only enhance outcomes and provide more stakeholders who want to be a part of the planned change. Otherwise, enthusiasm for projects may deteriorate rapidly, and what was initially recognized as a need or gap may become lost in the shuffle. All projects and their design should have solid supporting evidence and be guided by sound methods with rigor, keeping in mind the strategy and ultimate deliverables. Transparency cannot be emphasized enough with any project plan, design, implementation, and dissemination of outcomes. From a project's inception through its end point, remaining open and communicating progress engenders the spirit of ownership necessary for the final outcomes of the value-based project to be readily adopted by programs.

▶ Skills and Tools as Contributors to Meaningful Projects

In the fast-paced, ever-changing healthcare landscape, a plethora of skills and tools are needed throughout the life cycle of a project, but especially quality improvement ones. Envisioning a future state where the path forward can readily be recognized and followed by others is a deliberate action that leads to meaningful projects and supports their sustained management. The ability to manage the delicate dance of leading, engaging, and inspiring others toward greatness is one of the many skills needed by a project designer and manager. Investment in skill development and core competencies for project planning and management is central to shaping business outcomes in all industries, but especially health care. Applying human factors engineering in health care allows one to gain the knowledge needed to examine human behavior and interaction with others or with their surroundings and apply information for greater efficacy (Carayon & Wood, 2010; Gosbee & Anderson, 2003). Human factors engineering can further assist both the novice and expert project planner and manager in gaining insight into processes quickly and being able to initiate actions for course correction, as applicable.

The skills and tools needed for success with a project include an array of critical techniques and approaches. While there is no singular set of skills and tools that guarantees success, some options are mutually beneficial to individuals and organizations. The process for instilling these skills and tools into practice requires first understanding each and then linking it to goals and measurable, sustainable outcomes. Examples of skills and tools will be provided in this text, keeping in mind none is necessarily better than—or a replacement for—another.

Throughout an improvement project, keeping activities focused on the customers is important, especially when the organization depends on those customers for revenue and the majority of its market share. When customers are satisfied, loyalty is preserved and repeat business occurs. For example, if a manager requests the development of a quality improvement project that will increase customer satisfaction, it is important to first understand customer needs and expectations (understanding gleaned through the assessment process) and then to communicate those needs and expectations throughout the organization, while measuring value and reporting results.

Every project requires a designated leader to establish the direction of and ultimate goal for the project. While there may be informal leaders, the project leader should possess the skills needed to create and maintain the environment where others engage in meeting the project's goal. Creating opportunities to inspire others and involve them in both the current project and future projects is a mark of transformational leaders, who continually encourage and recognize others' contributions.

Being an effective communicator will engage others and provide the leverage necessary to initiate and complete projects in an expeditious fashion. However, this outcome will not occur without the ability, awareness, and sensitivity to address cultural differences in today's highly diverse workforce. All individuals process information differently due to their different cultural backgrounds and beliefs. Being aware and sensitive can facilitate progress on projects (Saxena, 2014; Seibert, Trejo, & Zimmerman, 2002).

Planning and organizational skills, such that one can assimilate information from various assessment processes and break down information into discrete parts, can set the stage for effective ongoing management of the project. Individual creativity may flourish when these skills are applied to organize outcomes for dissemination.

▶ Managing Projects and Teams in a Virtual Environment

One of the great rewards of technology is the opportunity to have global project team members contribute remotely. Project managers can leverage the strengths and talents of multiple individuals that match the project plan, strategy, and desired outcomes. As Porter-O'Grady and Malloch (2015) explain, teams are small systems and often mirror the complexity in other levels of the larger system. The effectiveness and performance of a project team, whether virtual or not, are contingent upon a combination of attributes and skill sets. These personal assets include individual competence, interpersonal skills, flexibility, accommodation, creativity, strong work ethic, and a focus on outcomes, to name a few. If the team has no identified purpose or end point, there is no meaning to the work to be accomplished. Projects may fail or yield limited outcomes that are not sustainable, and future virtual teams may be considered suspect.

As the moral compass for the virtual team, the leader should bring gentle diplomacy to bear in the discourse with staff, managers, stakeholders, and/or distractors. In particular, it is the virtual team leader's responsibility to defend the project and virtual team by shielding the overarching goal from distractors (Sturmberg & Martin, 2012). Adaptability becomes pivotal to success and is often more important than anticipation in such an environment.

Managing a virtual team can be rewarding as well as challenging. Virtual Hires (2014) identified nine guidelines that apply when selecting and managing individuals and teams in virtual environments:

1. Perform a project evaluation. Project leaders must be knowledgeable about goals, tactics, and deliverables if they are to communicate effectively with prospective team members.

2. Determine the skill sets needed by team members. Match the skills of team members to the delegated tasks and mutually reach consensus on assignments. Leveraging individual strengths promotes measurable outcomes.

3. Identify and anticipate obstacles. Knowing what has been attempted previously to resolve a problem or opportunity can only benefit the present outcomes. Conversely, disregarding this information can mean a loss for the plan, as the strategy may actually require only a minor redesign or assignment of a team member with matching skills and competencies.

4. Constantly engage members and encourage bidirectional communication. Contact with virtual team members often is employed to verify needs for supervision and encouragement. Likewise, the team member can communicate successes and challenges encountered that require intervention.

5. Establish a timeline and milestones. Identify expectations and the schedule needed to move the project toward completion. Monitor progress at designated intervals. Share accomplishments with all virtual members and stakeholders.

6. Ensure individual team member accountability. Recognizing the importance of each individual member's investment in achieving the critical priorities of a specific project and their buy-in to the larger institutional performance is a critical success factor.

7. Be cognizant of cultural differences. Being aware and sensitive to the diversity of virtual team members is important to avoid conflicts and delays in completing assigned tasks.

8. Manage conflict and difficult team members. Avoiding a conflict will only perpetuate the issue and result in inefficiency of the individual and team function. Although crucial conversations may be difficult on a personal

level, they are valuable for resolution of identified issues that may create project paralysis.

9. Provide education and training. Just-in-time or accelerated learning techniques may be required to assure all team members are on the same page with respect to the project goal and strategies. Using practical application examples and techniques matched with evidence, flexibility, and innovative teaching strategies can strengthen project outcomes and create synergy among virtual team members.

Effective governance and ownership of any project is critical to success. A poorly articulated and organized management structure, overlapping roles and decision-making authority, and mismatched roles and team members can prevent a project from achieving any momentum or producing valuable outcomes. The designated leader is the guardian of a finite project, who is charged with creating the structure and practices needed to guide the plan forward and strategically align it with the enterprise's overall direction.

Virtual teams hold much promise in the healthcare arena, where changing reimbursement models and movement toward greater industry transparency have placed substantial pressure on organizations to deliver stronger performance and improved value. In the long term, this trend is expected to continue. In turn, current improvements and projects focused on cost and quality performance will impel healthcare organizations toward higher standards requiring visionary leaders and dedicated project teams positioned to meet the challenges facing the healthcare industry.

▶ Summary

- Planning successful projects requires a series of deliberate and purposeful activities and a well-developed budget that result in an attainable goal.
- Projects may be limited to the microsystem or may extend to the meso- and macrosystem level(s) within an organization or industry.
- Projects are finite in scope, whereas program management extends across a system or industry.
- Leadership is central to successful projects and their sustainability.
- Projects that include the goals of the Triple and Quadruple Aims goals will benefit both systems and stakeholders.
- Envisioning a futuristic state opens up avenues for changes in behavior and value-based project outcomes.
- Technology affords opportunities for global project team membership where talents are leveraged toward an achievable goal.

Reflection Questions

1. Reflect on your current work environment and identify how leaders within the organization impact project successes, sustained practice change, and spread of evidence.
2. Identify and discuss a technological advance that may assist you as a capstone project is developed and implemented. Which technology might help you evaluate the project's impact within a healthcare system?

3. Which attributes contribute to a virtual project team's success? How can you ensure positive changes and outcomes as the project leader?
4. You are tasked with developing a project budget. What are the primary components to include in the budget?

References

Billows, D. (2014). *Project plan template: How to create a project plan.* Retrieved from http://4pm.com/project-plan-template

Bloch, R. (2017). Advantages and disadvantages of a virtual workforce *The Hartford.* Retrieved from https://www.thehartford.com/business-playbook/in-depth/virtual-workplace-advantages-disadvantages

Bodenheimer, T., & Sinsky, C. (2014). From triple to quadruple aim: Care of the patient requires care of the provider. *Annals of Family Medicine, 12*(6), 573–576.

Carayon, P., & Wood, K. E. (2010). Patient safety: The role of human factors and systems engineering. *Studies in Health Teaching and Informatics, 153,* 23–46.

Centers for Medicare and Medicaid Services. (2010). *Affordable Care Act update: Improving Medicare cost savings.* Retrieved from http://www.cms.gov/apps/docs/aca-update

Crisp, N. (2010). *Turning the world upside down: The search for global health in the 21st century.* London, UK: RSM Press.

Finkler, S. A., Jones, C. B., & Kovner, C. T. (2013). *Financial management or nurse managers and executives* (4th ed.). St. Louis, MO: Elsevier.

Frist, B. (2016). From volume to value: Achieving bold change in our healthcare payment systems. *Forbes.* Retrieved from https://www.forbes.com/sites/billfrist/2016/06/30/from-volume-to-value-achieving-bold-change-in-our-healthcare-payment-systems/#349507349c82

Gosbee, J., & Anderson, T. (2003). Human factors engineering design demonstrations can enlighten your RCA team. *Quality Safe Healthcare, 12,* 119–121.

Harrin, E. (2015). *How to plan a project budget.* Retrieved from https://www.projectmanager.com/blog/how-to-plan-a-project-budget

Haughey, D. (2014). *Project planning a step by step guide.* Retrieved from http://www.projectsmart.com/articles/project-planning-a-step-by-step-guide.php

Institute for Healthcare Improvement (IHI). (2014). *The IHI Triple Aim.* Retrieved from http://www.ihi.org.Engage/Initiatives/TripleAIM/Pages/default.aspx

Institute of Medicine (IOM). (2001). *Crossing the quality chasm: A new health system for the 21st century.* Washington, DC: National Academy Press.

Juran, J. M. (1992). *Juran on quality by design.* New York, NY: Simon and Schuster.

Lewis, J. P. (2011). *Project planning, scheduling and control: The ultimate hands-on guide to bringing projects in on time and on budget* (5th ed.). New York, NY: McGraw-Hill.

Lighter, D. M. (2011). *Advanced performance improvement in health care.* Sudbury, MA: Jones & Bartlett Learning.

Merrifield, R. (2009). *Re-think.* Upper Saddle River, NJ: Pearson.

Peters, T. (1999). *The wow project.* San Francisco, CA: Fast Company. Retrieved from http://www.fastcompany.com/36831/wow-project

Plsek, P. E., & Greenhalgh, T. (2001). The challenge of complexity in healthcare. *British Medical Journal, 323,* 625–628.

Porter, M. E. (2010). What is value in health care? *New England Journal of Medicine, 363,* 2477–2481.

Porter-O'Grady, T., & Malloch, K. (2015). *Quantum leadership: Building better partnerships for sustainable health.* Burlington, MA: Jones & Bartlett Learning.

Project Management Institute. (2013). *A guide to project management body of knowledge (PMBOK guide)* (5th ed.). Newtown Square, PA: Author.

Robert Wood Johnson Foundation. (2014). *Time to act: Investing in the health of our children and communities. Recommendations from the Robert Wood Foundation Commission to Build a Healthier America executive summary.* Retrieved from http://www.rwjf.org

Saxena, A. (2014). Workforce diversity: A key to improve productivity. *Procedia Economics and Finance, 11,* 76–85.

Seibert, P. S., Trejo, L. S., & Zimmerman, C. G. (2002). A checklist to facilitate cultural awareness and sensitivity. *Journal of Medical Ethics, 28,* 143–146.

Steinwachs, D. M., & Hughes, R. G. (2008). Health services research: Scope and significance. In R. G. Hughes (Ed.), *Patient safety and quality: An evidence-based handbook for nurses* (Vol. 1, pp. 163–177). Rockville, MD: Agency for Healthcare Research and Quality.

Stratton-Berkessel, R. (2010). *Appreciative inquiry for collaboration skills: 21-system-based workshop.* Hoboken, NJ: John Wiley & Sons, Inc.

Sturmberg, J. P., & Martin, C. M. (2012). Leadership and transitions: Maintaining the science in complexity and complex systems. *Journal of Evaluation and Clinical Practice, 18,* 186–189.

Tuthill, J. M. (2014). *Practical project management for informatics! How to manage a project without losing your mind.* Presentation at API Annual Conference, Chicago, IL.

Virtual Hires. (2014). *15 tips for effectively mapping your virtual employee.* Retrieved from http://www.virtualhires.com/resources.cgi?file=15-tips-to-effectively-managing-your-virtual-employee

World Health Organization (WHO). (2008). *Closing the gap in a generation: Health equity through action on the social determinants of health. Commission on Social Determinants of Health.* New York, NY: World Health Organization.

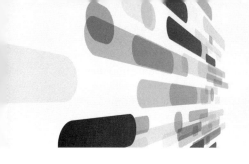

Case Exemplars

▶ ## Case Study 1

Guidepost for Students Selecting a Meaningful Capstone Project Topic

Jacqueline M. Lollar

As a former labor and delivery nurse in a teaching hospital and a current nurse educator, Sandy had always wanted to remain in the teaching and learning role. She began to recognize she had an excellent opportunity to advance her education. She had a great desire to earn a doctorate of nursing practice (DNP) degree and began discussing her options with mentors and colleagues. The university in which she was teaching had started a simulation program, and Sandy was involved in that program from the inception. She knew she wanted to incorporate human patient simulation and education into her capstone project.

When conducting literature searches related to simulation and nursing education, Sandy found that medication errors were a recurring theme. The first idea for her proposed capstone project was to implement simulated scenarios into the various nursing courses to decrease medication errors by student nurses and newly graduating novice nurses. That way, the students would be able to use their knowledge and skills in medication administration while causing no harm to live patients. If an error occurred, the students would be able to see the immediate reaction to a medication error.

After having numerous meetings with her faculty advisor and discussing the process for a needs assessment, Sandy completed a needs assessment at the institution. Upon the completion of the needs assessment, it was evident that the institution's faculty were already integrating medication administration in each simulated scenario. Sandy's idea was abandoned because medication administration was already a current practice at the College of Nursing. Additionally, with the guidance of her advisor, Sandy realized the project should have a more inclusive systems-change approach that would be better suited to a hospital setting. A change that could be incorporated into one unit in a hospital had the potential to change the entire culture of education throughout each department within a hospital.

After more meetings with her faculty advisor, Sandy began to explore the practices of area hospitals to determine the use of human patient simulation for educational purposes. One area hospital and labor and delivery unit shared a birthing simulator, Noelle, with another area hospital's labor and delivery unit. Each hospital had Noelle to use for a 6-month period of time. The labor and delivery nurse educator desperately wanted to utilize the simulator for educational purposes but had no expertise in its application. The nurse educator began explaining that the unit had numerous novice nurses and wanted them to participate in simulated scenarios focused on high-risk, low-volume obstetric patients. Additionally, she commented that The Joint Commission would be evaluating the hospital soon and the nursing staff was very weak in knowledge related to the National Patient Safety Goals (NPSGs). A shared belief between Sandy and the nurse educator working with the project was that competence in the discipline of nursing is paramount. Maintaining a level of competence is imperative for nursing staff to provide quality and safe patient care. However, competency is challenging to measure due to its many different components. The proposal of annual competencies, including NPSGs, was discussed at length with the nurse manager and nurse educator. At this time, buy-in for Sandy's capstone project was obtained.

Further conversations and meetings followed with the unit educator to determine the specific obstetric emergencies and NPSGs to be included in the annual competencies. The obstetric emergencies finally selected included fetal distress, amniotic fluid embolism, placental abruption, and postpartum hemorrhage. At the time, 10 NPSGs were in existence. Four NPSGs were selected for inclusion in the simulated scenarios based on common errors and staff needs: improve the accuracy of patient identification, improve the effectiveness of communication among caregivers, improve the safety of using medications, and accurately and completely reconcile medications across the continuum of care (The Joint Commission, 2008).

Sandy then began working closely with her faculty advisor to make the project both meaningful and sustainable. What theory would be the driving force for the project was a question approached first by the advisor. After conducting numerous literature searches and conversations with the faculty advisor, Sandy identified Dr. Patricia Benner's theory, from novice to expert, as the foundation for the project.

At this point, the DNP project had a theoretical basis and needed a model for change. The ACE Star Model of Knowledge Transformation was the model used for the quality improvement project. It enabled the discovery of knowledge to be implemented and transformed into practice. The ACE model consists of five cyclical phases: discovery, summary, translation, integration, and evaluation (Bonis, Taft, & Wender, 2007). While planning and implementing the project of using human patient simulation for annual competency validation for labor and delivery nurses, each phase of the ACE model was encountered.

Many variables were significant in planning for the implementation of each phase of the project. First, the institutional review board (IRB) had to approve the project to maintain protection for those subjects participating in the project. Although the project was one of quality improvement, protection of the participating subjects was an important aspect of the project, including future publication options. Approval by the IRB was required to be obtained before any steps in the implementation phases could begin at the institution. The information provided in the IRB application explained the purpose of the systems change project, as well as the risks and benefits to the participants. The faculty advisor played a major role in assisting and advising Sandy throughout the IRB approval process.

Information throughout the IRB application described the process of implementing the use of human patient simulation for annual competency validation. Although there were no anticipated risks associated with the quality improvement project, there was a minimal risk that staff might experience the normal anxiety typically associated with performance during the annual competency validations. Job security would not be compromised as a result of poor performance during the annual competencies. If a nurse did not perform at a level to meet the goal of 100% compliance, the staff nurse would be provided with review information and given more opportunities to repeat the simulated experience until the desired performance was achieved. However, the projected positive outcome would be an increase in the nursing staff's confidence in their management of obstetric emergencies, especially with high-risk, low-volume patients.

All labor and delivery nurses were required to participate in the annual competencies. Data collected for competency validation were kept confidential. The successful completion of the annual competencies would be stored in the nurse's personnel folder to maintain confidentiality. However, some level of privacy and confidentiality would be lost due to group participation, evaluation, and debriefing.

Approximately 60 labor and delivery nurses participated in the annual competency validation. The anticipated outcomes of the annual competency validations were positive. The goal of 100% compliance was met with each labor and delivery nurse. Human patient simulation provided an excellent learning opportunity for the labor and delivery nurses.

Continuous quality improvement was evident throughout the entire systems change process. The project provided benefits to both the hospital staff and their obstetric patients. Because the purpose of the project was one of quality improvement, the Institute of Medicine (IOM) aims were an important factor in the project, although each aim was not distinctly defined in this case. In general, the IOM aims include patient-centeredness, safety, effectiveness, efficiency, timeliness, and equity (Institute for Healthcare Improvement, 2009). Each aim was addressed in Sandy's quality improvement project, but the aim of safety was clearly a focal point throughout the implementation of the project. The project also incorporated evidence supporting human patient simulation as an effective learning tool for staff nurses. Experience is imperative for nurses to develop critical thinking skills and achieve competence. Once critical thinking skills and proficiency of psychomotor skills have been established, patient safety can be ensured.

The component of **sustainability** was in place from the initial meeting with the nurse manager and nurse educator. Many inquiries were made during the project regarding different strategies to incorporate into future simulated experiences for annual competencies. At the completion of the project, educational information and modules for the educator, as well as the staff nurses, were given to the unit educator for future use of the simulator. Information included in the modules dealt with pathophysiology, incidence, assessments, interventions, evidence-based practice articles, and case studies related to each of the obstetrical emergencies. Additionally, general information regarding The Joint Commission, accreditation, NPSGs, and elements of performance were included in the nurse's educational module.

Additional training and information were provided for educating the unit educator to maintain the sustainability of the project. Hands-on training, ranging from assembly of the simulator to moulaging to running scenarios, was provided to enable the unit educator to become proficient in using the simulator. A user manual was also developed for the unit educator, which included written and pictorial guides for future use.

Finally, several evaluation tools were developed and used for various aspects of the project and given to the nurse educator. One evaluation tool was developed to evaluate competence for each nurse with the obstetric emergencies as well as the chosen NPSG to be completed by the unit educator. Upon completion of the simulated scenarios, the staff nurses were given another evaluation tool to evaluate the experience during the scenarios.

Because it was well received by the institution and all of those involved, Sandy's project had great potential for sustainability. The labor and delivery unit educator planned to continue to use human patient simulation for annual competency validations. Also, other departments in the hospital were interested in using human patient simulation for various educational needs. One very exciting possibility was interprofessional use of human patient simulation, which was under discussion by the departments. The dissemination of findings, a very important factor, was also guided and supported by the faculty advisor. The project was presented at various conferences and introduced to surrounding hospitals.

The guidance by Sandy's advisor throughout the entire process of the quality improvement project and systems change was critical to the project's success. Without the direction and education provided by the advisor related to evidence, the project's theoretical basis, the project plan, the IRB process, analysis of data, and dissemination of the results, the project would not have had a solid foundation or the ability to maintain sustainability. Incorporating the use of human patient simulation for annual competency validation in a labor and delivery unit was a process that encompassed multiple strategic methods and various models. Obstetric emergencies are rare occurrences, but the nursing staff must be competent and maintain the ability to respond to them quickly and appropriately. The advisor, Sandy, the nurse educator, and the nurse manager firmly supported the use of human patient simulation for annual competency validation. The simulated scenarios assisted in bridging the gap between real patients and the learning opportunities for the labor and delivery nursing staff. Additionally, the incorporation of the National Patient Safety Goals into the simulated experiences assisted the organizations in maintaining compliance with The Joint Commission standards.

Reflection Questions

1. What are the benefits of completing a needs assessment prior to developing a clinical project? Consider which parts of a needs assessment may benefit you later as you engage in a clinical project.
2. How might a faculty advisor guide students throughout the clinical project?
3. How does completing the IRB process benefit the clinical project and its sustainability?

References

Bonis, S., Taft, L., & Wender, C. (2007). Strategies to promote success on the NCLEX-RN: An evidence-based approach using the ACE star model of knowledge transformation [Electronic version]. *Nursing Education Perspectives, 2*, 82–87.

Institute for Healthcare Improvement. (2009). *Science of improvement: Setting aims.* Retrieved from http://www.ihi.org/resources/Pages/HowtoImprove/ScienceofImprovementSettingAims.aspx

The Joint Commission. (2008). *National patient safety goals.* Retrieved from http://www.joint commission.org

▶ Case Study 2

Praxis: The Benefit to the Chief Nursing Officer as Projects Are Planned and Implemented

Wes Garrison

In any professional discipline, the overarching question of what guides practice is essential to understanding the framework within which practice occurs (Cody, 2013). Many factors influence the integration of theories and experiences that form the practice choices of an individual, and understanding the interrelation of those factors allows the individual to pursue knowledge, articulate practice, and communicate ideas more effectively. The process of integrating those theories and experiences is the underlying concept of praxis. As explained by Rolfe (1993), praxis is an ongoing, circular process of reflection in action whereby theory and practice continually inform, modify, and guide each other. Understanding the integration of informal theory and practice, a nurse executive can advance the profession and improve practice through a continual, circular process of reflection and action as projects are planned, implemented, and evaluated.

As the healthcare industry is evolving into a more technology-driven and resource-limited business model, the role of the nurse executive is becoming more business-focused. Certainly, clinical knowledge and skill are required for effective leadership of a nursing workforce, but a nurse executive also must understand how to direct quality care efficiently and communicate and collaborate effectively. Nurse executives must lead quality improvement initiatives to ensure cost-effective delivery of quality care (Carlson & Staffileno, 2013). Using relevant influences to form a nursing praxis to guide leadership allows for a structured, intentional approach to practice. By intentionally operating within the framework of a personal praxis, a nurse executive will continually improve leadership and advance the profession as projects evolve.

Ideological, Theoretical, and Ethical Influences

For a chief nursing officer, embracing an analytic approach as the primary philosophical viewpoint for practice allows for quantifying and measuring a variety of operational metrics. Based on empiricism, an analytic approach involves quantifiable data and definable results (Monti & Tingen, 1999). Empirical data allow a chief nursing officer to analyze relationships between quality improvement measures and cost-savings strategies. However, incorporating the continental approach to understand qualitative factors also is important for addressing less quantifiable aspects of nursing care and leadership (Monti & Tingen, 1999). Integrating both the analytic and continental approaches into leadership practice provides for a greater understanding of the nursing meta-paradigm and other relevant theoretical influences that guide projects throughout all phases.

From the broader framework of Fawcett's (1984) nursing meta-paradigm, Orem's (1991) Self-Care Deficit Nursing Theory (SCDNT) acts as instructive guide for teaching organizational goals for improving patient health and decreasing readmissions. Mc-Mahon and Christopher's (2011) middle-range theory for teaching the aesthetic skill of nursing presence is also an excellent guide for the continued education of nurses. In addition to nursing theories, the field of complexity science offers important guidance for practice in the explanation and understanding of complex adaptive systems.

Chief nursing officers must recognize the potential butterfly effect when even a small project or practice change is implemented (Florczak, Poradzisz, & Hampson, 2012).

Operating within an ethical framework is also imperative to effective and professional nursing practice. The theory of virtue ethics offers an appropriate context for professional practice. Focusing on the qualities of compassion, discernment, trustworthiness, integrity, and conscientiousness, virtue ethics provides a guideline for developing the qualities necessary for professionalism and for integrating those qualities into practice (Chism, 2013). In any leadership activity, a chief nursing officer must recognize the importance of instilling in nurses the ethical standards required for practice. By integrating the virtue ethics framework with the hospital-specific code of ethics, a nurse executive can communicate effectively to the nursing workforce the ethical expectations for practice. Keeping in mind the relevance of an ethics framework and its transparency is also pivotal as any project transpires.

Utilization of Framework: A Case Study

Understanding the benefit of a nursing praxis can be demonstrated by analyzing a chief nursing officer's (CNO) personal praxis (**FIGURE 1-1**) in the context of the phenomenon

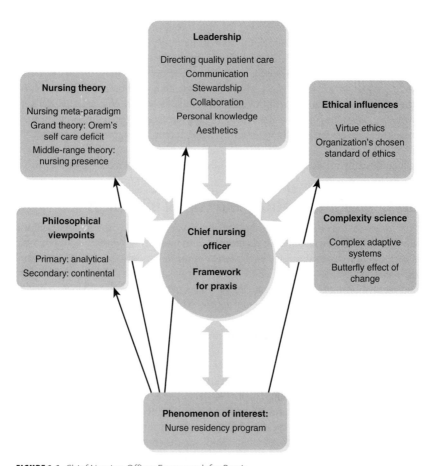

FIGURE 1-1 Chief Nursing Officer Framework for Praxis

of interest of nurse residency programs (NRPs) for new graduate registered nurses (RNs). Analyzing empirical data related to a high level of RN vacancies across the hospital, the CNO quantified the operational impact of the vacancies. Hospital volume was increasing, but the size of the RN workforce remained stagnant. Hospital policy required any RN being hired to have at least 2 years of RN experience. Available qualitative information revealed engagement and organizational loyalty within the existing RN workforce were decreasing due to the work demands caused by the vacancies.

Understanding the ethical obligation to provide quality care and the stewardship responsibilities for leading nursing practice, the CNO discerned the need to change the policy on hiring only experienced RNs. This change required implementing an NRP to address the needs of RNs transitioning to professional practice. In designing the NRP, the CNO stressed the importance of communicating the SCDNT for health promotion and the use of nursing presence theory to guide training simulations. Understanding the complex, adaptive nature of the hospital, the CNO anticipated a positive butterfly effect as the NRP eliminated vacancies, increased RN engagement, and improved the quality of care. As the NRP proceeded, the CNO planned to collect data on the effects of the NRP and determine which data will influence the CNO's praxis (Figure 1-1) for future guidance.

Reflection Questions

1. What are two benefits of praxis to nurses assigned to clinical and administrative roles?
2. How can you use the benefits of praxis to enhance your nursing knowledge and practice?

References

Carlson, E. A., & Staffileno, B. A. (2013). Establishing and sustaining an evidence-based practice environment. In M. A. Mateo & M. D. Foreman (Eds.), *Research for advanced practice nurses, from evidence to practice* (2nd ed., pp. 69–86). New York, NY: Springer.

Chism, L. A. (2013). The DNP graduate as ethical consultant. In L. A. Chism (Ed.), *The doctor of nursing practice* (2nd ed., pp. 179–212). Burlington, MA: Jones & Bartlett Learning.

Cody, W. K. (2013). Values-based practice and evidence-based care: Pursing fundamental questions in nursing philosophy and theory. In W. K. Cody (Ed.), *Philosophical and theoretical perspectives for advanced nursing practice* (5th ed., pp. 5–13). Burlington, MA: Jones & Bartlett Learning.

Fawcett, J. (1984). The meta-paradigm of nursing: Current status and future refinements. *Journal of Nursing Scholarship, 16*, 84–87. Retrieved from http://www.nursingsociety.org/Publication

Florczak, K., Poradzisz, M., & Hampson, S. (2012). Nursing in a complex world: A case for grand theory. *Nursing Science Quarterly, 25*, 307–312. doi:10.1177/0894318412457069

McMahon, M. A., & Christopher, K. A. (2011). Toward a mid-range theory of nursing presence. *Nursing Forum, 46*, 72–82. doi:10.1111/j.1744-6198.2011.00215.x

Monti, E. J., & Tingen, M. S. (1999). Multiple paradigms of nursing science. *Advances in Nursing Science, 21*, 64–80. Retrieved from http://journals.lww.com/advancesinnursingscience/pages/default.aspx

Orem, D. E. (1991). *Nursing: Concepts of practice* (4th ed.). St. Louis, MO: Mosby.

Rolfe, G. (1993). Closing the theory-practice gap: A model of nursing praxis. *Journal of Clinical Nursing, 2*, 173–177. doi:10.1111/j.1365-2702.1993.tb00157.x

▶ Case Study 3

Effective Virtual Teams

James L. Harris

To nurture innovation, creativity, and measurable outcomes, cultures are required that are supportive of virtual teams. Virtual teams offer opportunities for collaboration and generation of knowledge from different individual, organizational, and geographical perspectives. The Department of Veterans Affairs Office of Nursing Services is an excellent example of how virtual project teams are formed, work collaboratively to standardize standards of practice, spread innovation, and generate evidence (Thorne-Odem, Engstrom, Sommers, & Daly, 2015).

Virtual Field Advisory Committees (FACs), comprised of clinical experts and staff from numerous 152 Veterans Affairs Medical Centers, were formed, and a program coordinator provided national oversight. Each FAC identified key priority areas within the specialty area (gap analysis) and developed projects that focused on improving veteran care and providing tools and resources for staff in order to meet care needs. Outcome metrics were identified in order to track team effectiveness and outcomes that were aligned with national performance measures. FACs collaborated with multiple internal and external stakeholders, quality indicators, and competency-based assessment processes.

As indicated in this brief example, virtual teams provide value to organizations and patient care, and they engender staff engagement. While this was only one example, numerous healthcare organizations form virtual teams daily and collectively engage interprofessional teams to meet benchmarks and improve care.

Reflection Questions

1. How can you effectively contribute to a virtual team?
2. What are the key determinants of an effective virtual improvement team?

Reference

Thorne-Odem, S., Engstrom, C., Sommers, E., & Daly, A. (2015). Creating innovative models of nursing care. In C. Rick & P. B. Kritek (Eds.), *Realizing the future of nursing: VA nurses tell their story* (pp. 531–544). Washington, DC: U.S. Department of Veterans Affairs Veterans Health Administration.

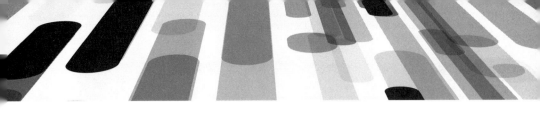

CHAPTER 2

Influences and Determinants of Quality Improvement Projects

Bettina Riley
James L. Harris

CHAPTER OBJECTIVES

1. Differentiate between quality improvement and research.
2. Identify historical influences, determinants, and unintended consequences associated with quality improvement projects.
3. Discuss the importance of legislation, health policy, and economics when designing quality improvement projects.
4. Explore the significance of organizational culture, social and environmental factors, and values and norms, to quality improvement projects.
5. Identify tools and methods that support meaningful quality improvement projects and evidence-based outcomes.

KEY TERMS

Design
Economics
Environment
Evidence-based
Health policy
History
Influences and determinants

Legislation
Organizational culture
Outcomes
Quality improvement projects and tools
Research
Value

ROLES	
Analyzer	Leader
Designer	Manager

PROFESSIONAL VALUES	
Ethics	Quality
Norms	Values

CORE COMPETENCIES	
Analysis	Evaluation
Assessment	Health policy knowledge
Designer	Innovation
Diversity	

▶ Introduction

The current healthcare system is driven by the need to respond to a rapidly changing **environment** and delivery of quality care. Healthcare quality is a universal marker that systems use to measure if care and desired **outcomes** are achieved (Batalden & Davidoff, 2014). The status quo is no longer acceptable. Current assumptions and processes must be challenged and replaced with robust improvements driven by measurable quality, safety, and **value**-based outcomes. **Influences and determinants** must be considered if improvements are valuable and sustainable within organizations. This requires positive engagement and actions by the entire healthcare team if systems of care are changed. Change must be based on clear expectations relevant to the situation and that foster relevant learning (Nelson et al., 2007). This is not a linear process, but a series of explorations resulting in meaningful outcomes (Moran, 2014).

This chapter focuses on influences and determinants of **quality improvement projects**. Threaded throughout the chapter are a differentiation of quality improvement projects and **research**; a discussion of historical influences, determinants, and unintended consequences related to improvement projects; relevance of **legislation**, **health policy**, and **economics**; and how **organizational culture** and environments influence outcomes of quality projects. Various tools and methods that support quality improvement projects are also provided in the chapter.

▶ Quality Improvement Projects Versus Research

Creating an environment receptive to change and **evidence-based** practice requires a series of purposeful actions and partnerships. Actions include various quality improvement projects that are led by interprofessional team members that culminate in practice change and sustainable outcomes. As project teams form, partnerships emerge and a common goal is established. Including researchers as an equal partner on the quality improvement project team is an asset, thus avoiding a waste of valuable resources. This creates venues for disseminating relevant information to the larger community (International Council of Nurses, 2012).

Often, individuals use language interchangeably. Differentiating between quality improvement and research proves beneficial in healthcare settings and can avoid barriers that lead to misunderstandings by improvement team members. For purposes of this chapter, the following definitions of quality improvement and research apply.

Quality improvement focuses on systems, processes, and functions associated with clinical quality, satisfaction, and cost outcomes. Meaningful quality improvement projects contribute to a better understanding of care processes through the application of knowledge. Research involves a process of systematic inquiry, whereby knowledge is developed, refined, and/or expanded. Research answers questions to develop knowledge grounded in a scientific method (Melnyk & Fineout-Overholt, 2005).

▶ Historical Influences, Determinants, and Unintended Consequences Associated with Quality Improvement Projects

History guides individual and group actions (Fairman & D'Antonio, 2013). This includes preparation and dissemination of policies, funding allocations, system improvements, and the **design** of quality improvement projects. Making sense and understanding the value of history when designing a quality project are invaluable. Historical data provide a lens to assess prior improvement attempts, processes, and variations in outcomes. History offers evidence that guides the work of quality improvement project teams and gives direction when choices are vague and lack basis.

Gaining insight into an organization's quality improvement project attempts and determinants of success is made easier when one considers three domains: process, structure, and outcomes. Process provides the context necessary to understand approaches that guide quality improvement project development and engagement of team members. Structure includes the specific elements that are most likely to have relevance and attain desired outcomes. Outcomes provide pathways for documenting efficacy and impacts of the project. Outcomes are further evident as project data are analyzed, communicated, and changes are adopted across the healthcare system.

Beyond the value of history and determinants of quality improvement project success are unintended consequences. Anticipating and managing the unintended consequences can be a daunting task. Unintended consequences extend beyond clinical effectiveness and include dismissal of evidence, social factors, financial impacts, and stakeholder partisanship. Evidence may be dismissed in certain regions, cultures, and groups. Evidence is moderated when controversy and differing opinions exist, limiting the development of a meaningful quality improvement project. Social environments may not be conducive to change based on current evidence. Evidence is desirable to ensure interventions are optimized, negative outcomes are minimized, and resources are used effectively. Realizing an immediate financial gain or incurring upfront costs may limit the full impact of a quality improvement project or its adoption. Partisanship among and between stakeholders may also affect buy-in of a quality improvement project, thus preventing or curtailing the design and initiation of projects that solidify quality, safety, and value-added outcomes.

Addressing and remaining cognizant of unintended consequences require the actions of all quality improvement team members. Advocating for the use of current evidence, interpreting the need for an evidence-based quality improvement project, and using available tools and resources are essential determinants of success.

▶ Importance of Legislation, Health Policy, and Economics When Designing Quality Improvement Projects

Demonstrating effectiveness in healthcare operations is required for sustainability in today's market. Doing more with less has resulted in organizations charging teams to design quality improvement projects that strengthen efficiency and accountability while achieving sustainable outcomes. Cost, quality, and access provide a basis for innovative improvement teams. Innovation is a critical value of alignment between the multiple forces affecting health care and decisions that follow (Porter-O'Grady & Malloch, 2015). As a quality improvement team begins to design a project, examining the impact of legislation and health policy offers insight into the demand to demonstrate effectiveness. Current legislation and health policy are grounded in evidence that informs budgets, management decisions, and strengthens accountability (Pew-MacArthur Foundation, 2015). Laws and public policies do not exist in a vacuum. Action taken in one domain may have unintended consequences in another domain while having synergistic, positive effects in yet another (Senterfitt, Long, Shih, & Teutsch, 2013). If quality improvement teams dismiss this reality, a disconnect will prevail, and the efficacy of project improvement project design, implementation, and outcomes will be jeopardized.

The convergence of team efforts forms a collective network of knowledge and facts as improvement projects are developed, implemented, and evaluated. Ruland (2010) concluded that facts increase decision quality, diminish errors, and strengthen the adoption of projects and outcomes.

Some of the most prominent healthcare organizations arise from the accumulation of knowledge. When a healthcare organization improves services, others adopt what works and benefit from its knowledge. The spread of this knowledge and its universal adoption result in situations that influence the economic outlook, sustainability, quality of services, and satisfied consumers.

The shift from volume-based to value-based care has required leaders to shift previous mental models of care to those that ensure advancement of the health of a nation (Centers for Medicare and Medicaid Services, 2013; U.S. Department of Health and Human Services, 2011). Likewise, quality improvement project design must balance innovation with value if a return on investment is realized. Using a cost-benefit model, project teams can create opportunities for practice change, whereby evaluation of outcomes is based on implementation with their fidelity to the original project design. This calls for project designs to reflect all work processes and activities subject to ongoing inquiry and reassessment (Porter-O'Grady & Malloch, 2015). Equally, incentives that balance innovation with value have sizeable implications for survival in the current healthcare arena. Incentives should be developed based on evidence-based economies, be fair, equitable, and have an intuitive appeal that benefits patient outcomes and system efficiency. Economics will continue to shape the landscape of health care and the design of quality improvement projects as reimbursement processes are reformed.

▶ Significance of Organizational Culture, Social and Environmental Factors, and Values and Norms to Quality Improvement Projects

There is no question that the culture of an organization, social and environmental factors, and values and norms affect the design, implementation, and adoption of quality improvement project outcomes. Universally, change in health care is driven by projects that result from errors, inefficiency, and survival instincts. Getting to the root cause of an issue becomes the foundation for a well-designed and executed quality improvement project.

Projects are advanced as leaders acknowledge the importance of context and culture. Assessing organizational culture is pivotal to planned change and adoption of improvements. Organizations that value quality improvement project team activities and their outcomes create windows of opportunity. As a result, the full potential of employees is realized, and care access, delivery, and efficiency are advanced. This requires moving from an organizational culture that blames others to adoption of a just culture (Khatri, Brown, & Hicks, 2009).

A just culture is an environment where an atmosphere of trusting, encouraging, and rewarding others for providing essential safety-related information occurs (Reason, 1997). A just culture addresses two areas: (1) the role of punitive sanction in the safety of the healthcare system and (2) the effects of a punitive sanction as a remedy for human error as a help or hindrance to safety efforts (Marx, 2001). With adoption of a just culture during the past decade, numerous advances in healthcare practices and operations have been achieved (Kennedy, 2016).

Social and environmental factors are important to consider for any quality improvement project team. These factors are the largest predictor of health outcomes and are influential in changing practices (Sentefitt et al., 2013). Health and health-related problems result from multiple factors. For example, factors such as educational level, employment, environment where individuals live and work, and support are primary determinants of health outcomes. As quality improvement teams design projects, remaining aware of these factors is essential if outcomes are realized (Mosadeghrad, 2014). Consider the current debate surrounding requirements for immunizing infants and preschoolers. Addressing the social and environmental factors related to immunizations requires others to interpret evidence, advocate for adherence, and align messages that are supportive of universal practices. Similarly, the adoption of quality improvement project findings can be impacted by social group acceptance and the environment targeted for change. Advocacy for change becomes paramount in these circumstances.

One's values and norms in society also influence quality improvement projects. If individuals or organizations have conflicting values associated with a project, the likelihood of the development or success is endangered. Societal norms also affect acceptance of a project and its outcomes. If the norm is to only adopt changes from one specific group, new projects and ideas are destined for disapproval or failure.

▶ Tools and Methods Supporting Evidence-Based Quality Improvement Projects

The idea that evidence-based quality improvement projects transform practice and advance quality is a strategic differentiator tool for sustaining a competitive edge (Mosadeghrad, 2014). Achieving equilibrium between practice and quality offers a regimen to ensure all evidence is available as quality improvement projects are developed and completed. However, this does not occur as a singular process but requires use of various tools and techniques that support meaningful quality improvement projects.

Identifying a problem is not enough. Problem identification leads to an improvement based on a process of analysis that is scientifically validated and a rigorous standardized methodological approach. Lloyd (2004) detailed the science underpinnings for all improvement as being grounded in the scientific method. Lloyd integrates the deductive (general to specific) and inductive (specific to general) phases of the scientific method, thus creating opportunities that support quality improvement projects. The information gained from the process is central to decision-making.

Another technique is using Force Field Analysis. Developed by Kurt Lewin (1946), this technique allows project teams to identify stakeholders and issues that may deter improvement processes. The technique also allows teams to identify supporting allies and create new scenarios for team building (International Council of Nurses, 2012).

Using performance indicators as a tool in determining what causes variation in outcome is fundamental to the work of quality improvement teams. Performance indicators inform policy makers, improve quality of care, identify poor performers, and provide consumer information. There are four primary reasons for variation in outcome: (1) differences in patient type, (2) differences in measurement, (3) chance, and (4) differences in quality care. While there are advantages to process and outcome indicators, explanations of variation limit the value of outcome measures. Conversely, process measures are more sensitive to measuring differences in quality of care and are easy to interpret (Marx, 2001).

James Reason's Swiss Cheese Model of a System (2008) offers quality improvement project teams another tool to identify latent or hidden failures in a system. Identifying failures in policies, institutional culture, team functions, individual competency, and technology often provides insight into an error and the needed corrective action.

A foundation approach, Plan-Do-Study-Act (PDSA) developed by W. Edwards Deming, is another valuable tool (Langley et al., 2009). This tool involves a circular motion and multiple interactions in an improvement cycle. *Plan* involves planning the change. *Do* is carrying out the change. *Study* includes analyzing results to determine what went wrong or was learned. *Act* involves adopting the change, abandoning it, or repeating the cycle (Deming, 1993).

Quality improvement project teams also use accreditation standards. The standards encompass three major areas:

1. *Patient-focused functions*: Rights, ethics, and responsibilities; provision of care, treatment, and services; medication management; and surveillance, prevention, and control of infection.

2. *Organizational functions*: Improving organizational performance; leadership; management of the environment of care; management of human resources; and management of information.
3. *Structures and functions:* Medical staff; nursing (The Joint Commission, 2004).

A systematic review is another tool commonly used by quality improvement project teams. It is a comprehensive approach to locating and synthesizing the evidence on an identified issue. Through an organized, transparent, and replicable process, initial issues are resolved (Littell, Corcoran, & Pillai, 2008). A scale of proposed benefit emerges, and the fit with an existing or proposed policy and consideration of potential for harm, ease of application, and enactment are possible.

Various statistical techniques offer advantages for quality improvement projects and teams and include measures of variability and central tendency, tests of significance, and correlation. Data analysis tools such as brainstorming, nominal group technique, run charts, control charts, flowcharts, a fishbone cause-and-effect diagram, histograms, and Pareto charts also have significant value. Descriptions and examples of each are commonly found in management and statistics textbooks.

Two final tools include political competence and savvy. Political competence is the ability to assess and translate the impact of change (Longest, 1988). Equally important is political savvy. Political savvy is the ability to cut across organizations, culture, and global boundaries when establishing priorities and actions (DeLuca, 1999). Possessing political competence and strategic foresight is a requisite skill needed by quality improvement project teams as health care is increasingly more regulated, unpredictable, and global (Habegger, 2009).

▶ Summary

- The status quo in health care is no longer acceptable. Current assumptions and processes must be challenged and replaced with robust quality improvement projects driven by measurable quality, safety, and value-based outcomes.
- Influences and determinants must be considered if improvements are valuable and sustainable within organizations. This requires positive engagement and actions by the entire care team if systems of care are changed and sustainable.
- Quality improvement focuses on systems, processes, and functions associated with clinical quality, satisfaction, and cost outcomes.
- Research involves a process of systematic inquiry, whereby knowledge is developed, refined, and/or expanded.
- History guides individual and group actions. Making sense and understanding the value of history when designing a quality project is invaluable. Historical data provide a lens to assess prior improvement attempts, processes, and variations in outcomes.
- Process provides the context necessary to understand approaches that guide quality improvement project development and engagement of team members. Content includes the specific elements that are most likely to have relevance and attain desired outcomes. Outcomes provide pathways for documenting the efficacy and impacts of the project.
- Cost, quality, and access provide a basis for innovative improvement teams.

- Current legislation and health policy are grounded in evidence that informs budgets, guides management decisions, and strengthens accountability.
- The spread of this knowledge and its universal adoption result in situations that influence the economic outlook, sustainability, quality of services, and satisfied consumers.
- The culture of an organization, social and environmental factors, and values and norms affect the design, implementation, and adoption of quality improvement project outcomes.
- A just culture is an environment where an atmosphere of trusting, encouraging, and rewarding others for providing essential safety-related information occurs.
- Social and environmental factors are the largest predictor of health outcomes and are influential in changing practices.
- Values and norms in society influence the outcomes of quality improvement projects.
- Evidence-based quality improvement projects transform practice and advance quality. Such projects are a strategic differentiator tool for sustaining a competitive edge.
- Achieving equilibrium between practice and quality offers a regimen to ensure all evidence is available as quality improvement projects are developed and completed.
- Multiple tools, methods, and techniques exist that offer quality improvement project teams to identify latent or hidden failures in a system.

Reflection Questions

1. When developing a quality improvement project or proposal, what are the primary considerations to ensure success and practice change outcomes are sustained?
2. Select a quality improvement project. What are the tools and methods that will assist you throughout the process?
3. How would you differentiate between structure, process, and outcome indicators? How may each be incorporated in a quality improvement proposal?

References

Batalden, P. B., & Davidoff, F. (2014). What is "quality improvement" and how can it transform healthcare? *Quality Safe Health Care, 16*(1), 2–3.

Centers for Medicare and Medicaid Services. (2013). *Bundled payments for care improvement (BPCI) initiative: General information.* Retrieved from http://innovation.cms.gov/initiatives/bundled-payments

DeLuca, J. R. (1999). *Political savvy: Systematic approaches to leadership behind the scenes.* Berwyn, PA: EBG.

Deming, W. E. (1993). *The new economics.* Cambridge, MA: MIT Press.

Fairman, J., & D'Antonio, P. (2013). History counts: How history can shape our understanding of health policy. *Nursing Outlook, 61,* 346–352.

Habegger, B. (2009). Strategic foresight: Anticipation and capacity to act. *CSS Analyses in Security Policy.* Retrieved from http://works.bepress.com/beathatter/19

International Council of Nurses. (2012). *Closing the gap: From evidence to action.* Geneva, Switzerland: Author.

Kennedy, B. (2016). Toward a just culture. *Nursing Management, 46*(6), 13–15.

Khatri, N., Brown, G.D., & Hicks, L. L. (2009). From a blame culture to a just culture in health care. *Health Care Management Review, 34*(4), 312–322.

Langley, G. J., Moen. R. D., Nolan. K. M., Nolan, T. W., Norman, C. L., & Provost, L. P. (2009). *The improvement guide* (2nd ed.). San Francisco, CA: Jossey-Bass.

Lewin, K. (1946). Force field analysis. In J. E. Jones & J. Pfeiffer (Eds.), *The 1973 annual handbook for group facilitators* (pp. 111–113). San Diego, CA: University Associates.

Littell, J. H., Corcoran, J., & Pillai, V. (2008). *Systematic reviews and meta-analysis.* New York, NY: Oxford University Press.

Lloyd, R. (2004). *Quality health care: A guide to developing and using indicators.* Sudbury, MA: Jones and Bartlett Publishers.

Longest, B. (1998). Managerial competence at senior levels of integrated delivery systems. *Journal of Healthcare Management, 17,* 299–307.

Marx, D. (2001). *Patient safety and the "just culture": A primer for health care executives.* New York, NY: Columbia University.

Melnyk, B. M., & Fineout-Overholt, E. (2005). *Evidence-based practice in nursing and healthcare.* Philadelphia, PA: Lippincott Williams & Wilkins.

Moran, K. (2014). Setting the state for the doctor of nursing practice scholarly project. In K. Moran, R. Burson, & D. Conrad (Eds.), *The doctor of nursing practice scholarly project. A framework for success* (pp. 3–14). Burlington, MA: Jones & Bartlett Learning.

Mosadeghrad, A. M. (2014). Factors influencing healthcare service delivery. *International Journal of Health Policy Management, 3*(2), 77–89.

Nelson, E. C., Batalden, P. B., Homa, K., Godfrey, M. M., Campbell, C., Headrik, L. A., . . . Wasson, J. H. (2007). Creating a rich information environment. In E. C. Nelson, P. B. Batalden, & M. M. Godfrey (Eds.), *Quality by design. A clinical microsystems approach* (pp. 178–196). San Francisco, CA: John Wiley & Sons, Inc.

Pew-MacArthur Foundation. (2015). *Legislating evidence-based policymaking. A look at state laws that support data-driven decision-making.* Retrieved from http://www.pewtrusts.org/en/projects /pew-macarthur-results-first-initiative

Porter-O'Grady, T., & Malloch, K. (2015). *Quantum leadership: Building better partnerships for sustainable health.* Burlington, MA: Jones & Bartlett Learning.

Reason, J. (1997). *Managing the risks of organisational accidents.* London, U.K.: Ashgate Publishing.

Reason, J. (2008). *The human contribution: Unsafe acts, accidents, and heroic recoveries.* Burlington, VT: Ashgate Publishing.

Ruland, C. (2010). Translating evidence into practice. In W. L. Holzmer (Ed.), *Improving health through nursing research.* Geneva, Switzerland: International Council of Nurses.

Senterfitt, J. W., Long, A., Shih, M., & Teutsch, S. M. (2013). How social and economic factors affect health. *Social Determinants of Health, 1,* 1–22.

The Joint Commission. (2004). *The Joint Commission press kit.* Retrieved from http://www .jointcommission.org/NewsRoom/PressKits

U.S. Department of Health and Human Services. (2011). *Hospital value-based purchasing program.* Retrieved from http://www.cms.gov/Outrearch-and-Education/Medicare-Learning-Network -MLN/MLNProducts/downloads/Hospital_VBPurchasing_Fact_Sheet_ICN907664.pdf

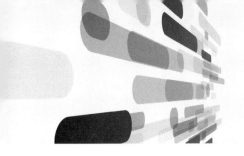

Case Exemplars

▶ Case Study 1

Increasing Therapeutic Communication Skills Using Behavioral Simulation

Bettina Riley

Based on an identified need to improve therapeutic communication skills in an undergraduate nursing course, behavioral simulation was used. This was based on one component of a team-based learning (TBL) strategy, the use of active learning versus passive learning techniques to increase knowledge (Michaelsen, Parmelee, McMahon, & Levine, 2008). Parmelee (2010) purports that TBL improves knowledge and critical thinking among nursing students.

The behavioral simulation session focused on a specific patient safety goal (i.e., depression with suicide risk) and was linked to suicide risk assessment, cited as a major patient safety goal by The Joint Commission (2017). The behavioral scenario emphasized the importance of suicide risk assessment building on the establishment of a trusting, therapeutic nurse–patient relationship. The simulation experience utilized standardized patients trained in a prepared scenario prior to the event. Training emphasized depression criteria with suicidal ideations. The participants included 96 undergraduate nursing students. The students were involved in a pre-simulation educational TBL activity on suicide and suicide risk assessment. Next, individual students interviewed a standardized patient for purposes of completing a psychiatric assessment focused on suicide risk. Students were rotated through eight simulation rooms, and students and peers videotaped the assessment for future review. Debriefing sessions, led by psychiatric mental health faculty, followed each behavioral simulation. The purpose of debriefing was expression of feelings and exploration of benefits for clinical application. Student and faculty evaluation of the team-based learning, simulation, and debriefing experiences has been very positive. Positive evaluations by students centered on the ability to have a safe practice zone for acquiring assessment skills, particularly in sensitive-topic areas—over 93% of nursing students expressed more confidence in the ability to assess suicide risk, and over 90% of the students found that the standardized patient scenario, combined with the TBL, was helpful and effective. Anecdotal findings from faculty included comments that when students went to community and inpatient clinical sites after the behavioral simulation, they exhibited greater confidence and knowledge in clinical assessment of suicide risk and therapeutic communication skills.

Reflection Questions

1. What are other components of team-based learning that can be developed to enhance learning and competency development in baccalaureate nursing students?
2. In what ways can team-based learning activities be evaluated?

References

Michaelson, L. K., Parmelee, D. X., McMahon, K. K., & Levine, R. E. (2008). *Team-based learning for health professions education. A guide to using small groups for improving learning.* Sterling, VA: Stylus Publishing, LLC.

Parmelee, D. X. (2010). Team-based learning: Moving forward in curriculum innovation: A commentary. *Medical Teacher 32*(2), 105–107.

The Joint Commission. (2017). National patient safety goals effective January 2017. Behavioral health care accreditation program—Goal 15. *Behavioral Health Care: National Patient Safety Goals*, 1–4. Retrieved from https://www.jointcommission.org/assets/1/6/NPSG_Chapter_BHC_Jan2017.pdf

▶ Case Study 2

Increasing Access to Mental Health Treatment Using the Internet: A Quality Improvement Project Proposal

Jennifer Anne Blalock

Background

While the Affordable Care Act (ACA) continues to face challenges, it nevertheless presented an opportunity to improve mental health treatment. Underfunded and underutilized mental health treatment is desperately in need of change. The age of technology and widespread use of the Internet present a new avenue for access and mental health care delivery. Rural populations will be able to receive more efficient and timely care.

Han et al. (2015) report that in 2012, approximately 9.6 million Americans above the age of 17 were diagnosed with a serious mental illness (SMI). Depression alone affects 35 million Americans over 65 years of age (Golden & Vail, 2014). Richards et al. (2015) acknowledge that depression is among the leading causes of disability worldwide, creating a significant economic burden, and the gap in treatment for depression is estimated to be 56.3%. Several contributing reasons are identified, including stigma associated with mental health treatment, physical and financial access to care, and availability of services. Costs of treatment for patients with an SMI are significant. However, the cost of preventive care, such as therapy and medication management, is considerably less than the cost of inpatient care or criminalization of those left untreated. According to the Stensland, Watson, and Grazier (2012), the average hospital's cost of care delivery was highest for patients with Medicare and lowest for those uninsured. To use two common diagnoses, treatment for depression ranged from $6,990 for 8.4 days to $3,616 for 4.4 days, and alcohol use disorder treatment ranged from an average of $5,908 for 6.2 days to $4,147 for 3.8 days. Hoban (2013) compared the cost of mental health treatment, including medication management and outpatient services, for those on Medicaid to the cost of arrest and involvement in the criminal justice system; those arrested cost the government an average of $95,000 during the study period compared to $68,000 for those not arrested and channeled into mental health treatment. While treating mental illness is expensive, the cost of NOT treating mental illness is more so. It is with this and similar studies in mind that a proposal to increase outreach and provide new access to care is presented.

Addressing the Treatment Gap

As healthcare providers in the United States struggle to meet the needs of mental health consumers, the use of the Internet, or eMental Health, has become an attractive option. Batterman et al. (2015) reviewed four models of eHealth implementation in the community and found that all four were effective in the treatment of depression. ePrograms demonstrated several advantages to patients, particularly in the availability of services and increased access. By providing a common point of access, patients were able to locate both free and paid services in the community, allowing for self-referral without initial contact with a primary care physician (PCP). Handley et al. (2014) provide further support for Internet-based mental health treatment, noting that such services make treatment options available to rural communities that would otherwise lack access to a mental health provider. Their results indicate that eHealth is as effective in treating mental health disorders as face-to-face contact and reduces the anxiety some patients experience in these interactions. Not only do web-based programs increase care access, but they also improve the timeliness of treatment, as there is no wait time and adherence to normal business hours is not necessary.

Proposed Project Implementation

Psychiatric providers will have the option of utilizing web-based services in several ways: continuation of already established, ongoing therapy; as a component of aftercare treatment upon completion of intensive services; provision of a 24-hour crisis line to direct new patients to web-based services as determined appropriate by telephone triage. More patients can be treated, including those without access to transportation or those hesitant to seek face-to-face treatment. Use of eServices will be established on a sliding scale and fee-for-service copays based on insurance providers, providing additional revenue. Free services can also be included, funded by endowments or special purpose funds.

A business model with three layers will be developed creating an eMental Health program: the patient layer (patients or payers that use the service), the operational service layer (operations, equipment, management, training, legal, billing, reimbursement), and the infrastructure layer (the telecommunication itself, including Internet and wireless services). Implementation of eMental Health services can be integrated as part of the already-existing services as part of a behavioral health program, which encompasses two residential facilities as well as outpatient care.

For successful delivery of this relatively new concept, a development team will be necessary. This team will incorporate a variety of practitioners, including psychiatrists, medical physicians, nurses, and social workers, as well as a clinic manager, hospital administrator, and information technology (IT) development and support staff. Practice guidelines will be developed (hours of operation, policies specific to Web interactions, etc.). Although these can run parallel to and include those already in place for existing psychiatric care facilities, attention to Internet-related confidentiality must be considered. A new policy will be written. IT staff are critical in the development of web-based program components, with input from direct-care users, and in identifying costs and limitations. Design of the program will be done within the existing computer programs, thus reducing the cost of new software and licenses. Training time for staff already familiar with the platform will be reduced. Having an electronic medical record operational will strengthen the success of the eMental Health program. Once fully operational, with outcome measures that support continued use of an eMental Health program, additional delivery methods can be considered and employed, such as smartphone applications. Nicholas, Fogarty, Boydell, and Christensen (2017) found, in a study of individuals diagnosed with bipolar disorder, that the mobility of smartphone apps further increased accessibility, was cost-effective, and allowed more client anonymity.

Evaluation

The structure of this proposal includes the use of computers and Wi-Fi, both public, such as those available in libraries, and those located within the patient's home. Staff involved in the program will utilize technology provided in on-site facilities. However, some home access may be granted as determined by the program director. Additional staffing will be needed to address the increased referrals anticipated from the implementation of eServices. The numbers required will likely increase over time as use of the program broadens. Use will be monitored to determine how many new staff are required. Initially, patient interactions will be managed with current staff plus one new psychiatrist, two family psychiatric nurse practitioners (FPNPs), and two additional psychiatric registered nurses. Web-based client interactions will be a portion of total patient contacts, the majority of which will remain face-to-face. Web visits will be billed at a lower cost than face-to-face visits, with some patients receiving pro bono services.

Process measures of the eHealth program will include tracking referrals and comparing data collected at three points: prior to program initiation, during the implementation phase, and later, during the sustainability phase. It is important to know not only if the number of referrals increased but also the number of patient contacts within the website. User-friendliness is a critical measure for web-based interactions and should be assessed regularly to ensure ease of use by patients and staff. The use of patient-satisfaction surveys will be critical in determining this aspect of the program. These can be mailed for completion or "attached" at the end of an Internet session. Staff surveys will be utilized to determine areas that work well and those that require modification.

More important than use alone, the program needs to be effective and increase access to mental health services. The outcome of the program will be determined by comparing the number of patient psychiatric contacts before initiation of web-based services to those after implementation. This should be calculated at 6-month intervals for the first 18 months. The number of crisis inpatient admissions must also be compared to determine if web-based services produced a reduction in admissions by providing more access to psychiatric care by 50%. Pre and post evaluations by patients will be conducted to gain an understanding of what patients found helpful and what needs to be improved. In addition, pre and post symptom assessment will be completed to determine effectiveness.

The return on investment for eMental Health services should not be anticipated as a black-and-white, financially based result. Initial investment costs could take several years to demonstrate cost savings related to decreased inpatient admissions or revenue created by increased patient contacts. Rather, the main purpose of the investment is enhancement of care quality. Swensen et al., (2013) note four instances of poor care quality that can be improved with this program: overuse care, defective care, inefficient care, and underuse care. By broadening effective psychiatric services, all of these can be addressed among individuals with mental health diagnoses. Overuse of inpatient psychiatric crisis admissions can be reduced, more effective and efficient care can be provided, and access to care can be increased. While, over time, these changes have potential to reduce costs to Medicare, Medicaid, and private insurance, the reason to adopt the program is not financial gain. This initiative is recommended to improve quality of care, not produce a financial return. By investing more in patients, genuine care and concern for patients' health outcomes will be evident, contributing to an improved reputation in the community and, ultimately, gaining increased credibility and potentially more patient flow and revenue as a result.

Conclusion

Web-based services provide a new opportunity for growth in the initial and ongoing treatment of patients with mental health diagnoses. While use of this form of treatment remains in the introductory phase, the capacity to further the development of this approach is promising. Providing mental health care to a larger portion of the population by significantly increasing access, particularly for patients hesitant to engage face-to-face, those in rural communities, or those simply lacking transportation, is a valid rationale for the proposal. The timeline may vary, but it is anticipated to take approximately 18 months from the first team meeting to a full live rollout. Financially, the return on investment cannot yet be clearly defined, although in time, reduced cost for services and increased revenue are anticipated. Mental health is a global issue and one that remains underfunded and underrecognized. With the inception of web-based services, the chance to become an innovator and a leader in the rapidly changing world of health care is possible. More importantly, many more patients can benefit from mental health treatment that was previously out of reach.

Reflection Questions

1. Consider that the mental health clinic where you are employed has experienced a 40% face-to-face missed-appointment rate. What options would you propose to the program director and why?
2. Reflect on a change in an organization. What are key considerations that resulted in the success or failure associated with the change, and why? What would you propose to improve the change?

References

Batterman, P. J., Sunderland, M., Calear, A. L., Davey, C. G., Christensen, H., Teesson, M., & Krouskos, D. (2015). Developing a roadmap for the translation of e-mental health services for depression. *Australian & New Zealand Journal of Psychiatry*, *49*, 776–784. http://dx.doi.org/10.1177/0004867415582054

Golden, R. L., & Vail, M. R. (2014). The implications of the Affordable Care Act for mental health care. *Journal of American Society on Aging*, *38*, 96–103. Retrieved from www.asaging.org/generations-journal-american-society-aging

Han, B., Gfroerer, J., Kuramoto, J., Ali, M., Woodward, A., & Teich, J. (2015). Medicaid expansion under the Affordable Care Act: Potential changes in receipt of mental health treatment among low-income nonelderly adults with serious mental illness. *American Journal of Public Health*, *105*, 1982–1989. Retrieved from https://www.apha.org/publications-and-periodicals/american-journal-of-public-health

Handley, T. W., Kay-Lambkin, F. J., Inder, K. J., Attia, J. R., Lewin, T. J., & Kelly, B. J. (2014). Feasibility of internet-delivered mental health treatments for rural populations. *Social Psychiatry and Psychiatric Epidemiology*, *49*, 275–282. http://dx.doi.org/10.1007/s00127-013-0708-9

Hoban, R. (2013, July 1). NC state study shows why it costs less to treat mentally ill than incarcerate them. *North Carolina Health News*. Retrieved from http://www.northcarolinahealthnews.org/2013

Nicholas, J., Fogarty, A. S., Boydell, K., & Christensen, H. (2017). The reviews are in: A qualitative content analysis of consumer perspectives on apps for bipolar disorder. *The Journal of Medical Internet Research*, *19*, 1–18. http://dx.doi.org/10.2196/jmir.7273

Richards, D., Timulak, L., O'Brien, E., Hayes, C., Sharry, J., & Doherty, G. (2015). A randomized controlled trial of an internet-delivery treatment: Its potential as a low-intensity community intervention for adults with symptoms of depression. *Behaviour Research and Therapy*, *75*, 20–31. http://dx.doi.org/10.1016/j.brat.2015.10.005

Stensland, M., Watson, P. R., & Grazier, K. L. (2012). An examination of costs, charges, and payments for inpatient psychiatric treatment in community hospitals. *Psychiatric Services*, *63*, 666–671. http://dx.doi.org/10.1176/appi.ps.201100402

Swensen, S. J., Dilling, J. A., McCarty, P. M., Bolton, J. W., & Harper, C. M. (2013). The business case for health-care quality improvement. *Journal of Patient Safety*, *9*, 44–52. Retrieved from www.journalpatientsafety.com

CHAPTER 3

Implementation Science and Team Science: The Value for Projects

Clista Clanton
Linda Roussel

CHAPTER OBJECTIVES

1. Provide an overview of implementation and team science.
2. Discuss a variety of implementation science theoretical frameworks.
3. Identify key characteristics for successful teamwork through implementation science.
4. Describe implications of project management through an implementation science lens.

KEY TERMS

Implementation science
Interprofessional Education Collaborative (IPEC)
Knowledge translation

National Center for Advancing Translational Science (NCATS)
Science of Team Science (SciTS)
Translational science

ROLES

Healthcare researcher

Healthcare team member

PROFESSIONAL VALUES

Evidence-based practice   Teamwork
Patient-centered care

CORE COMPETENCIES

Cultural competency and   Interprofessional collaboration
   awareness   Resilience
Emotional intelligence   Shared problem-solving
Flexibility   Team building skills

▶ Introduction

The complexity of health care has led to the development of disciplines such as translational, implementation, and team sciences. While interrelated and complementary, each discipline is distinct. This chapter will focus primarily on implementation and team sciences, yet it is helpful to place all three disciplines into context, as the development of each is directly related to specific needs and events within research and healthcare systems. An examination of how each area has developed gives a snapshot in time to some of the challenges healthcare professionals currently face in their day-to-day roles within practice settings, as well as ways to meet these challenges. Implications for project planning and management will be described.

It is estimated that it takes 17 years for research evidence to make an impact on clinical practice (Morris, Wooding, & Grant, 2011), which highlights the significant time lags in the conversion of basic science into practices that benefit patients. This process of conversion is what is referred to as "translation," and each phase of the translational research process has activities which contribute to these time lags, including securing financing in the form of grants, receiving approvals from institutional review boards (IRBs), conducting clinical trials, presenting and publishing research results, and developing practice guidelines. Furthermore, there are different phases in the translational research process, and the activities contributing to these time lags may occur in more than one phase:

T1: involves processes that bring ideas from basic research through early testing in humans

T2: involves the establishment of effectiveness in humans and clinical guidelines

T3: primarily focuses on implementation and dissemination research

T4: focuses on outcomes and effectiveness in populations

T0: involves research, such as genome-wide association studies, that wraps back around to basic research (Fort, Herr, Shaw, Gutzman, & Starren, 2017)

The term *translational research* first appeared in health science literature in the early 1990s, and given the relative newness of the field of **translational science**, it makes sense that formal definitions continue to evolve. **National Center for Advancing Translational Science (NCATS)** of the National Institutes of Health (NIH) currently

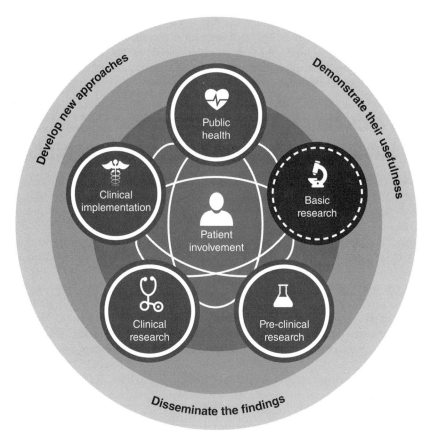

FIGURE 3-1 NCATS Translational Science Spectrum (*National Center for Advancing Translational Sciences at the National Institutes of Health*).

describes a Translational Science Spectrum (**FIGURE 3-1**), which "represents each stage of research along the path from the biological basis of health and disease to interventions that improve the health of individuals and the public. The spectrum is not linear or unidirectional; each stage builds upon and informs the others." Patient involvement is considered a critical feature of all the stages of the translation process (NCATS, 2015a). The Clinical and Translational Science Awards (CTSA) Program operates under the leadership of NCAT to support a national network of medical research institutions known as "hubs." In 2017, it was estimated that 57 medical research institutions in the United States would receive CTSA Program funding, with the hubs collaborating at both the local and regional level to develop and promote training, research tools, and processes designed to get more evidence into practice as quickly as possible and to make a positive impact on patient care (NCATS, 2015b, c).

The T3 and T4 phases of the translational research process introduce us to **implementation science**, which is "the study of methods to promote the adoption and integration of evidence-based practices, interventions and policies into routine health care and public health settings" (Fogarty International Center, 2017). The synthesis of research findings into digestible formats for inclusion in systematic reviews, practice guidelines, and other evidence-based resources is one of the strategies to help healthcare professionals implement relevant evidence into clinical practice (Straus, Tetroe, & Graham, 2009).

There are multiple conceptual frameworks that provide structure to the implementation of evidence into practice, including the Promoting Action on Research Implementation in Health Sciences (PARiHS), the Consolidation Framework for Implementation Research (CFIR), the Knowledge to Action Framework (KTA), and the Aims, Ingredients, Mechanism, Delivery framework (AIMD). Brief overviews of these frameworks follows.

▶ Promoting Action on Research Implementation in Health Sciences (PARiHS)

Promoting Action on Research Implementation in Health Sciences (PARiHS) is a multidimensional framework designed to represent the complexity of the change processes involved in implementing research into practice and includes three elements: evidence, context, and facilitation. In the PARiHS framework, evidence includes research, clinical experience, patient experience, and local data/information. The PARiHS framework is outlined as: SI = f (E, C, F) Specifically, SI is successful implementation; E denotes evidence; C relates to context; F is facilitation and f denotes the function of the change process. In the PARiHS, the factor of evidence, context and facilitation consists of sub-elements that can be scored (rated) on a scale from low to high. According to researchers, high ratings on each factor are more likely to produce successful implementation results (Kitson et al., 1998; Kitson et al., 2008).

Implementation processes are likely to be more successful when research and clinical and patient experiences are located toward high. For research, high includes studies that are rigorous and have received consensus. High for clinical experiences are those that have been made explicit and verified via critical reflection, critique, and debate. Patient experience is considered at a high level when patient preferences have been used as part of the decision-making process. For local data and information to be considered high, they should have been systematically collected and evaluated.

Context in the PARiHS framework refers to the environment or setting where people receive health care as well as the environment or setting in which the proposed changes are to be implemented. Successful implementation of evidence into practice is influenced by three broad themes: culture, leadership, and evaluation. Organizations that create learning cultures are potentially able to facilitate change more easily, as attention is paid to individuals, group processes, and organizational systems. Transformational leaders are those who are able to transform cultures and create contexts that are more conducive to the integration of evidence into practice. They do this through inspiring staff to have a shared vision and by establishing clear roles, effective teamwork, and organizational structures. Evaluation is a key component in the environment, as measurement generates evidence on which to base practice and demonstrates if changes to practices have been successful.

Facilitation in the PARiHS framework refers to the process of enabling or making easier the implementation of evidence into practice. This is achieved by an individual with the appropriate role, skills, and knowledge who acts as a facilitator to help individuals, teams, and organizations apply evidence into practice. High facilitation in the PARiHS framework is holistic (sustained partnerships, developmental, adult learning approaches, high intensity/limited coverage) and with an appropriate level of facilitation, whereas low facilitation is more task oriented (episodic contact, practical/technical help, didactic approach to teaching, low intensity/extensive coverage) and would correspond to either absent or inappropriate facilitation (Rycroft-Malone, 2004).

In order for the PARiHS conceptual heuristic to become a truly useful and integrated framework for practitioners of implementation science, three areas have been identified that need further work: conceptual development, empirical testing and refinement, and the development of reliable measures to diagnose and evaluate readiness to change and the effectiveness of that change within an organization (Kitson et al., 2008). Subsequent studies have reinforced the need for development in these three areas and have suggested other issues to consider, such as the role that individuals play in the implementation process. To that end, the integrated or i-PARiHS has been proposed as a more integrated approach. In addition to the key constructs of evidence, context, and facilitation, a new construct has been suggested: the recipient, or the people who are affected by and influence implementation at both the individual and collective team level. This new construct recognizes the importance that groups or teams of individuals have in influencing the adoption of evidence into practice. The i-PARiHS also makes a distinction between the inner context of the immediate local setting versus the outer context of the wider health system that the organization is a part of, including the policy, social, regulatory, and political infrastructures surrounding the local context. The facilitation construct is also positioned as the active ingredient of implementation, with networks of novice, experienced, and expert facilitators who help structure the process while engaging and managing relationships with key stakeholders as well as identifying and negotiating the barriers to implementation within their settings (Harvey & Kitson, 2016).

Consolidation Framework for Implementation Research

The lack of consistent terminology and definitions in implementation theories as well as no one theory containing all of the key constructs needed for successful implementation has been identified as a problem in the science of implementation, leading to the development of the Consolidated Framework for Implementation Research (CFIR; CFIR Research Group, n.d.). This meta-theoretical framework contains the common constructs identified from published implementation theories and is designed to embrace, rather than replace, the already-existing significant research related to implementation science. The CFIR's goal is to help advance the field by providing consistent taxonomy, terminology, and definitions and to allow researchers to select the constructs from the CFIR that are the most relevant for their particular setting and needs.

The CFIR is composed of five major domains which interact with each other to influence the effectiveness of implementation. **TABLE 3-1** briefly describes the domains, but more comprehensive information on each is available at http://cfirguide.org /constructs.html. These constructs are meant to provide a beginning foundation for understanding implementation as well as provide a guide for formative evaluations of intervention studies and programs. The CFIR can also be used to organize and promote the synthesis of implementation research findings and studies, as the constructs included in the framework can be used to more clearly explain the concepts in a consistent manner across studies (Damschroder et al., 2009). Damschroder et al. (2009) provide commentary on fostering health services research implementation (findings into practice) aligning the CFIR framework for advancing the science.

Knowledge-to-Action (KTA) Framework

The Knowledge-to-Action (KTA) Framework is meant to help conceptually clarify key elements involved with moving knowledge into action. Recognizing that the multiple

TABLE 3-1 Consolidated Framework for Implementation Research Constructs

Construct		Short Description
I. Intervention Characteristics		
A	Intervention Source	Perception of key stakeholders about whether the intervention is externally or internally developed.
B	Evidence Strength and Quality	Stakeholders' perceptions of the quality and validity of evidence supporting the belief that the intervention will have desired outcomes.
C	Relative Advantage	Stakeholders' perception of the advantage of implementing the intervention versus an alternative solution.
D	Adaptability	The degree to which an intervention can be adapted, tailored, refined, or reinvented to meet local needs.
E	Trialability	The ability to test the intervention on a small scale in the organization and to be able to reverse course (undo implementation) if warranted.
F	Complexity	Perceived difficulty of implementation, reflected by duration, scope, radicalness, disruptiveness, centrality, and intricacy and number of steps required to implement.
G	Design Quality and Packaging	Perceived excellence in how the intervention is bundled, presented, and assembled.
H	Cost	Costs of the intervention and costs associated with implementing the intervention, including investment, supply, and opportunity costs.
II. Outer Setting		
A	Patient Needs and Resources	The extent to which patient needs, as well as barriers and facilitators to meet those needs, are accurately known and prioritized by the organization.
B	Cosmopolitanism	The degree to which an organization is networked with other external organizations.
C	Peer Pressure	Mimetic or competitive pressure to implement an intervention, typically because most or other key peer or competing organizations have already implemented, or are in a bid for, a competitive edge.

Construct		Short Description
D	External Policy and Incentives	A broad construct that includes external strategies to spread interventions, including policy and regulations (governmental or other central entity), external mandates, recommendations and guidelines, pay-for-performance, collaboratives, and public or benchmark reporting.
III. Inner Setting		
A	Structural Characteristics	The social architecture, age, maturity, and size of an organization.
B	Networks and Communications	The nature and quality of webs of social networks and the nature and quality of formal and informal communications within an organization.
C	Culture	Norms, values, and basic assumptions of a given organization.
D	Implementation Climate	The absorptive capacity for change; shared receptivity of involved individuals to an intervention; and extent to which use of that intervention will be rewarded, supported, and expected within their organization.
1	Tension for Change	The degree to which stakeholders perceive the current situation as intolerable or needing change.
2	Compatibility	The degree of tangible fit between meaning and values attached to the intervention by involved individuals; how those align with individuals' own norms, values, and perceived risks and needs; and how the intervention fits with existing workflows and systems.
3	Relative Priority	Individuals' shared perception of the importance of the implementation within the organization.
4	Organizational Incentives and Rewards	Extrinsic incentives such as goal-sharing awards, performance reviews, promotions, and raises in salary, and less tangible incentives such as increased stature or respect.
5	Goals and Feedback	The degree to which goals are clearly communicated, acted upon, and fed back to staff, and alignment of that feedback with goals.

(continues)

TABLE 3-1 Consolidated Framework for Implementation Research Constructs *(continued)*

	Construct	Short Description
6	Learning Climate	A climate in which (a) leaders express their own fallibility and need for team members' assistance and input; (b) team members feel that they are essential, valued, and knowledgeable partners in the change process; (c) individuals feel psychologically safe to try new methods; and (d) there is sufficient time and space for reflective thinking and evaluation.
E	Readiness for Implementation	Tangible and immediate indicators of organizational commitment to the decision to implement an intervention.
1	Leadership Engagement	Commitment, involvement, and accountability of leaders and managers with the implementation.
2	Available Resources	The level of resources dedicated for implementation and ongoing operations, including money, training, education, physical space, and time.
3	Access to Knowledge and Information	Ease of access to digestible information and knowledge about the intervention and how to incorporate it into work tasks.
IV. Characteristics of Individuals		
A	Knowledge and Beliefs About the Intervention	Individuals' attitudes toward, and value placed on, the intervention as well as familiarity with facts, truths, and principles related to the intervention.
B	Self-Efficacy	Individuals' belief in their own capabilities to execute courses of action to achieve implementation goals.
C	Individual Stage of Change	Characterization of the phase an individual is in as they progress toward skilled, enthusiastic, and sustained use of the intervention.
D	Individual Identification with Organization	A broad construct related to how individuals perceive the organization and their relationship with and degree of commitment to that organization.
E	Other Personal Attributes	A broad construct to include other personal traits such as tolerance of ambiguity, intellectual ability, motivation, values, competence, capacity, and learning style.

Construct		Short Description
V. Process		
A	Planning	The degree to which a scheme or method of behavior and tasks for implementing an intervention are developed in advance, and the quality of those schemes or methods.
B	Engaging	Attracting and involving appropriate individuals in the implementation and use of the intervention through a combined strategy of social marketing, education, role modeling, training, and other similar activities.
1	Opinion Leaders	Individuals in an organization who have formal or informal influence on the attitudes and beliefs of their colleagues with respect to implementing the intervention.
2	Formally Appointed Internal Implementation Leaders	Individuals from within the organization who have been formally appointed with responsibility for implementing an intervention as coordinator, project manager, team leader, or other similar roles.
3	Champions	Individual dedicated "to supporting, marketing, and driving through an implementation, overcoming indifference or resistance that the intervention may provoke in an organization" (Powell et al., 2015, pg. 9).
4	External Change Agents	Individuals who are affiliated with an outside entity who formally influence or facilitate intervention decisions in a desirable direction.
C	Executing	Carrying out or accomplishing the implementation according to plan.
D	Reflecting and Evaluating	Quantitative and qualitative feedback about the progress and quality of implementation accompanied by regular personal and team debriefing about progress and experience.

terms used in the KTA field were only contributing to confusion, the creators of the KTA Framework reviewed multiple interdisciplinary planned action theories about the process of change and developed a framework focused on the concepts of knowledge creation and the action cycle that leads to the implementation or application of knowledge. Knowledge creation is represented as a funnel and consists of the knowledge or research types used in health care. As the knowledge moves through the funnel, it becomes more synthesized or refined (synopses, practice guidelines, clinical care pathways) and feasibly more usable by stakeholders. Action cycles contain the activities needed for knowledge implementation and are dynamic, influencing each other as well as being influenced by the knowledge creation phases. Commonalities within the various planned action theories reviewed are represented by the following phases:

- Identify a problem that needs addressing
- Identify, review, and select the knowledge or research relevant to the problem
- Adapt the identified knowledge or research to the local context
- Assess barriers to using the knowledge
- Select, tailor, and implement interventions to promote the use of knowledge
- Monitor knowledge use
- Evaluate the outcomes of using the knowledge
- Sustain ongoing knowledge use (Graham et al., 2006)

The KTA Framework is one of the most frequently cited conceptual frameworks for **knowledge translation** but is being used in practice with varying degrees of completeness and theory exactness when integrated into an implementation process. Many of the studies that have utilized the KTA framework were conducted in Canada, no doubt a reflection of the association of the KTA Framework with the Canadian Institutes of Health Research and the subsequent adoption by Canadian research funding organizations. These studies reported and gave examples of how the KTA Framework was integral to the design, delivery, and evaluation of their implementation activities, with enactment of the KTA Framework ranging from informing to full integration, indicating a flexibility of use for local needs and circumstances (Field, Booth, Ilott, & Gerrish, 2014).

Aims, Ingredients, Mechanism, Delivery (AIMD)

To address the issue of multiple terminologies and frameworks within the field of implementation science, an international collaboration of scholars met in 2012 to develop a simplified framework to describe interventions that promote and integrate evidence into health practices, systems, and policies. Their goal was to create a "meta-framework" that would accommodate the use of existing frameworks in the field and was thus designed to be "terminology agnostic." To that end, the working research group was comprised of members from the fields of quality improvement, evidence synthesis, policy, information science, public health, patient safety, and behavior change. The framework developed as a result of these initial efforts was composed of four components: (1) Intended targets, or the intended effects of the intervention and/or its beneficiaries; (2) Active ingredients, or the critical components that define the intervention and are required to initiate change; (3) Causal mechanisms, or the proposed pathways or policies by which an intervention will effect change; and (4) Mode of delivery or application, or the ways in which active ingredients are applied.

The original framework went through a validation project and further refinement over the next 3 years, resulting in the validated and revised version of the simplified framework version 1, now called the AIMD framework (**TABLE 3-2**). The AIMD framework still contains the four original components, but the concepts and associated descriptions were made more simple and clear. As a result, Intended Targets became AIMS, Active Ingredients became Ingredients, Causal Mechanisms became Mechanisms, and Mode of Delivery or Application became Delivery.

TABLE 3-2 The AIMD Framework

Component	Description
Aims	What do you want your intervention to achieve and for whom?
Ingredients	What comprises the intervention?
Mechanism	How do you propose the intervention will work?
Delivery	How will you deliver the intervention?

Bragge, P., Grimshaw, J. M., Lokker, C., & Colquhoun, H. (2017). *AIMD: A Validated, Simplified Framework Of Interventions To Promote And Integrate Evidence Into Health Practices, Systems, and Policies. BMC Medical Research Methodology, 17* (38). Retrieved from https://doi .org/10.1186/s12874-017-0314-8

The creators of AIMD believe it can serve as a framework for effective communication between team members of implementation interventions as well as serve as a guide for the development of intervention designs and reporting toolkits (Bragge, Grimshaw, Lokker, & Colquhoun, 2017).

Selecting the appropriate implementation framework to guide local projects may be confusing, and some recommendations to help improve the process include using methods such as concept mapping, group model building, conjoint analysis, and intervention mapping (Powell et al., 2017). Checklists for identifying the determinants of practice, including one tool with a focus on behavior change in health professionals, are available and may prove useful for those who are designing, conducting, evaluating, or reporting implementation projects (Flottorp et al., 2013). For those who are involved in implementation research, the Standards for Reporting Implementation Studies (StaRI) initiative developed a 27-item checklist that provides a guideline for the transparent and accurate reporting of implementation studies. The StaRI standards are registered with the EQUATOR Network (http://www.equator-network.org), where the checklist is available as a download (Pinnock et al., 2017).

Value of Implementation and Team Science for Sustainable Clinical Projects

Team science applies conceptual and methodological approaches from multiple disciplines and health professions in order to address complex clinical problems. While there is a growing emphasis on interprofessional training for health professions students to prepare them for team-based clinical practice, training for researchers who are team or interprofessionally based has traditionally been lacking. It is also increasingly being recognized that truly effective patient care requires a combination of both interprofessional medical practice and transdisciplinary scientific knowledge, which necessitate clinical practice guidelines that take into account team-based care and that integrate knowledge from multiple disciplines (Begg et al., 2014; Croyle, 2008). The NIH recognizes the importance of cross-disciplinary science, in which team members with training and expertise in different fields work together to combine or integrate their perspectives in a single research endeavor, which is seen as a promising approach to accelerate both scientific innovation and the translation of scientific findings into effective policies and practices (National Cancer Institute, n.d.). The National Institute for Mental Health (NIMH) has made team science a priority and has designed a 2-year training institute in mental health implementation science called the Implementation Research Institute (IRI). Both mentoring and collaboration are emphasized in the training program, and an analysis of the IRI has demonstrated a significant impact of the mentoring relationships on future scientific collaborations, as evidenced by increases in grants, presentations, and publications produced by IRI attendees and their mentors in a post-training 2-year time span (Luke, Baumann, Carothers, Landsverk, & Proctor, 2016).

A team science academic–industry hybrid model, the multidisciplinary translational team (MTT), is a combination of several team types adapted for an academic setting and includes an interprofessional group of scientists who are working together to solve a common translational problem. The CTSA has provided support for MTTs in the form of infrastructure and team development training, including orientation meetings to the CTSA for team members, assistance with producing team and individual objectives and tasks, the development of team leadership councils which functioned as a peer mentoring network, and hosting a team-building workshop. An evaluation of MTTs showed four different team type trajectories, which indicates the need for team specific interventions in the areas of leadership and resources to help them reach their maximum potential: (1) teams with traditional leadership; (2) teams focused on basic science; (3) stable, high-functioning teams with junior project managers; and (4) teams with inexperienced leaders. The teams that were identified as having effective team processes developed interdisciplinary concepts and publications that most likely would not have happened without the interaction between the team members (Wooten et al., 2015).

The **Science of Team Science (SciTS)** is a rapidly growing field which has the potential to positively impact both translational and implementation science and to improve health care. Interprofessional teams are not limited to just translational or research teams, as the complexity of providing optimal patient care within our modern healthcare system necessitates well-functioning teams comprised of healthcare providers, administrative leaders, support staff, patients, industry, and community agencies/members. The composition of these teams will fluctuate depending on the task at hand, the need for different types of expertise, access to resources/personnel, or any other number of variables inherent in healthcare organizations. Many of the skills identified in the SciTS literature apply as much to clinical teams as they do to research teams, and strengthening teamwork has been identified as a top priority for improving health care, especially when it comes to patient safety (Clancy & Tornberg, 2007). The argument can be made that "soft skills" are integral for effective collaboration and team functioning and may not have received adequate emphasis in the health sciences curriculum during professional training. Many of these soft skills are addressed in the **Interprofessional Education Collaborative (IPEC)** Core Competencies for Interprofessional Collaborative Practice, which focus on four domains: (1) values/ethics: work with individuals of other professions to maintain a climate of mutual respect and shared values; (2) roles/responsibilities: use the knowledge of one's own role and those of other professions to appropriately assess and address the needs of healthcare patients and to promote and advance the health of populations; (3) interprofessional communication: communicate with patients, families, communities, and professionals in health and other fields in a responsive and responsible manner that supports a team approach to the promotion and maintenance of health and the prevention and treatment of disease; and (4) teams/teamwork: apply relationship-building values and the principles of team dynamics to perform effectively in different team roles to plan, deliver, and evaluate patient/population-centered care and population health programs and policies that are safe, timely, efficient, effective, and equitable (IPEC, 2017). Each domain includes sub-competencies that further identify the skills and actions needed to achieve the IPEC core competencies. These skills and actions can also be thought of in broader categories, such as cultural and diversity awareness, emotional intelligence, strategic thinking, conflict resolution, persuasion, resilience, flexibility, and the ability to inspire moral- and competence-based trust, and have been identified for contributing to the ability to successfully collaborate with others in a variety of disciplines (Gibert, Tozer, & Westoby, 2017).

Data from interviews with NIH researchers who were part of five teams that ranged from successful (defined as teams that developed a reasonable level of cohesiveness and were able to pursue their missions) to groups that ended because of conflict indicate that the following characteristics contribute to an effective team: effective leadership, self and other awareness, established trust among team members, open communication strategies, shared expectations, clear definition of roles and responsibilities, a shared vision, appropriate recognition and credit given to team members, allowing for disagreement while mitigating conflict, learning each other's languages, and enjoying the science and working together (Bennett, Gadlin, & Levine-Findley, 2010) Trust has been identified as one of the most critical elements for successful teams and therefore should not be left to chance. Specific steps that can be taken to proactively build trust within teams include having explicit conversations where partnership expectations are discussed, on what the roles within the team will be, on how information/data/resources will be shared, on how decisions will be made, and on how disagreements or conflicts will be handled (Bennett & Gadlin, 2012).

Key contributing characteristics for successful teamwork such as the development of a common understanding of both the roles of team members and the structure of the work have been referred to as a shared mental model (SMM) (Canon-Bowers, Salas, & Converse, 1993). The SMM construct, as it relates to clinical teamwork and health professions learners to date, has not been well defined, with interventions to foster or measure SMM in clinical teams being not well represented in the published literature (Floren et al., 2017). There are a variety of tools which can be used to measure teamwork, however, including those that measure the teamwork of individuals working within teams, the teamwork of teams as a whole, and those that assess both individuals and teams. One of the more well-known ones is the TeamSTEPPS Teamwork Attitudes Questionnaire, which is designed to assess the teamwork attitudes, knowledge, and skills of learners who have gone through the TeamSTEPPS curriculum (Agency for Healthcare Research and Quality, 2016). Another validated tool that has been associated with improved patient outcomes is the Team Climate Inventory, which was originally designed to measure a team climate for innovation using five scales related to: (1) Participative safety; (2) Support for innovation; (3) Vision; (4) Task orientation; and (5) Social desirability (Anderson & West, 1996). Over 70 unique tools designed to quantitatively measure teamwork in an internal medicine setting have been identified in the literature, indicating no lack of resources for those looking to assess teamwork in their local setting (Havyer et al., 2014). Clearly, the behavior of healthcare professionals and healthcare organizational culture are key variables that impact the quality of patient care and the sustainability of clinical projects. Staying abreast of research findings in the fields of both implementation and team science can equip those who are part of clinical care teams or who are conducting quality improvement and research projects with strategies and tools that will better enable successful outcomes.

▶ Implications for Project Planning and Management

Understanding implementation science models and the various tools and strategies for moving evidence into true practice and sustained improvement provides the "next steps" in the uptake of evidence-based practice. Common language and terminology provide a beginning to the effective spread and scale-up of successful projects. Incorporating the science of team science, working together as interprofessional teams, can also be facilitative in the process. Being able to "diagnose" teamwork attitudes, knowledge, and skills of learners through the use of assessment tools will be important to a starting point in developing a shared mental model. Trust is a cornerstone of team success and positive outcomes. Evaluation of the structure, processes, and outcomes of the actual implementation and the team's effectiveness advances real-time improvement and sustainability for population health management.

▶ Summary

- Strategies to address the real-world needs of patients and the providers who care for them are the impetus behind translational, implementation, and team science in health care.
- National networks such as PCORnet, the National Patient-Centered Research Network, are actively working to improve health and health care by fostering faster, less expensive, and more powerful ways to conduct observational and experimental clinical effectiveness research (CER) studies, utilizing strong partnerships between patients, clinicians, and health systems via 33 partner networks and a Coordinating Center (Patient-Centered Outcomes Research Institute, 2016).
- Advances in the fields of implementation science and team science are identifying effective strategies for healthcare providers to take the evidence produced from these research studies and apply them to improve the health of patients in their local settings.
- While the challenges of working in multidisciplinary or interprofessional teams can be great, the benefits of increased opportunities for new scientific knowledge, mentorship, and innovation can provide great rewards that will benefit patients, practice settings, organizations, and healthcare systems.

Reflection Questions

1. What role do you see for yourself in the more efficient and timely implementation of evidence into practice to help improve the health of patients?
2. What are some of the characteristics essential to fostering a productive team environment?
3. How can you contribute to an organizational culture that promotes and rewards collaboration?
4. Consider your last project. How did you use (or could use) an implementation model and team science principles?

Learning Activities

Identify a program or clinical project that would benefit from the structure provided by an implementation science theory or framework. Which theory or framework would you use and why?

What characteristics or strategies do you believe would best work for promoting team cohesiveness in your practice environment? How would you go about improving teamwork in your environment?

References

Agency for Healthcare Research and Quality (AHRQ). (2016, May 20). *TeamSTEPPS* Retrieved from https://www.ahrq.gov/teamstepps/index.html

Anderson, N., & West, M. (1996). The Team Climate Inventory: Development of the TCI and its applications in teambuilding for innovativeness. *European Journal of Work and Organizational Psychology*, 5(1), 53–66.

Begg, M. D., Crumley, G., Fair, A. M., Martina, C. A., McCormack, W. T., Merchant, C., . . . Umans, J. G. (2014). Approaches to preparing young scholars for careers in interdisciplinary team science. *Journal of Investigative Medicine: The Official Publication of the American Federation for Clinical Research*, 62(1), 14–25. https://doi.org/10.231/JIM.0000000000000021

Bennett, L., Gadlin, H., & Levine-Findley, S. (2010). *Team science and collaboration: A field guide*. Bethesda, MD: Department of Health and Human Services. Retrieved from https://ccrod.cancer.gov/confluence/download/attachments/47284665/TeamScience_FieldGuide.pdf

Bennett, L. M., & Gadlin, H. (2012). Collaboration and team science: From theory to practice. *Journal of Investigative Medicine: The Official Publication of the American Federation for Clinical Research*, 60(5), 768–775. https://doi.org/10.2310/JIM.0b013e318250871d

Bragge, P., Grimshaw, J. M., Lokker, C., & Colquhoun, H. (2017). AIMD—A validated, simplified framework of interventions to promote and integrate evidence into health practices, systems, and policies. *BMC Medical Research Methodology*, 17, 38. https://doi.org/10.1186/s12874-017-0314-8

Canon-Bowers, J., Salas, E., & Converse, S. (1993). Shared mental models in expert team decision-making. In N. J. Castellan (Ed.), *individual and group decision making: Current issues* (pp. 221–246). Hillsdale, NJ: Lawrence Erlbaum Associates.

Clancy, C. M., & Tornberg, D. N. (2007). TeamSTEPPS: Assuring optimal teamwork in clinical settings. *American Journal of Medical Quality: The Official Journal of the American College of Medical Quality*, 22(3), 214–217. https://doi.org/10.1177/1062860607300616

Croyle, R. T. (2008). The National Cancer Institute's transdisciplinary centers initiatives and the need for building a science of team science. *American Journal of Preventive Medicine*, 35(Suppl-2), S90–93. https://doi.org/10.1016/j.amepre.2008.05.012

CFIR Research Team. (n.d.) *Consolidated Framework for Implementation Research (CFIR)*. Retrieved from http://cfirguide.org/constructs.html

Damschroder, L. J., Aron, D. C., Keith, R. E., Kirsh, S. R., Alexander, J. A., & Lowery, J. C. (2009). Fostering implementation of health services research findings into practice: A consolidated framework for advancing implementation science. *Implementation Science*, 4, 50. https://doi.org/10.1186/1748-5908-4-50

Field, B., Booth, A., Ilott, I., & Gerrish, K. (2014). Using the Knowledge to Action Framework in practice: A citation analysis and systematic review. *Implementation Science*, 9, 172. https://doi.org/10.1186/s13012-014-0172-2

Floren, L. C., Donesky, D., Whitaker, E., Irby, D. M., Ten Cate, O., & O'Brien, B. C. (2017). Are we on the same page? Shared mental models to support clinical teamwork among health professions learners: A scoping review. *Academic Medicine*. Advance online publication. https://doi.org/10.1097/ACM.0000000000002019

Flottorp, S. A., Oxman, A. D., Krause, J., Musila, N. R., Wensing, M., Godycki-Cwirko, M., . . . Eccles, M. P. (2013). A checklist for identifying determinants of practice: A systematic review and synthesis of frameworks and taxonomies of factors that prevent or enable improvements in healthcare professional practice. *Implementation Science: IS*, 8, 35. https://doi.org/10.1186/1748-5908-8-35

Fogarty International Center. (2017, July 27). *Implementation science information and resources.* Retrieved from https://www.fic.nih.gov/researchtopics/pages/implementationscience.aspx

Fort, D. G., Herr, T. M., Shaw, P. L., Gutzman, K. E., & Starren, J. B. (2017). Mapping the evolving definitions of translational research. *Journal of Clinical and Translational Science, 1*(1), 60–66. https://doi.org/10.1017/cts.2016.10

Gibert, A., Tozer, W. C., & Westoby, M. (2017). Teamwork, soft skills, and research training. *Trends in Ecology & Evolution, 32*(2), 81–84. https://doi.org/10.1016/j.tree.2016.11.004

Graham, I. D., Logan, J., Harrison, M. B., Straus, S. E., Tetroe, J., Caswell, W., & Robinson, N. (2006). Lost in knowledge translation: Time for a map? *The Journal of Continuing Education in the Health Professions, 26*(1), 13–24. https://doi.org/10.1002/chp.47

Harvey, G., & Kitson, A. (2016). PARIHS revisited: From heuristic to integrated framework for the successful implementation of knowledge into practice. *Implementation Science : IS, 11.* https://doi.org/10.1186/s13012-016-0398-2

Havyer, R. D. A., Wingo, M. T., Comfere, N. I., Nelson, D. R., Halvorsen, A. J., McDonald, F. S., & Reed, D. A. (2014). Teamwork assessment in internal medicine: A systematic review of validity evidence and outcomes. *Journal of General Internal Medicine, 29*(6), 894–910. https://doi.org/10.1007/s11606-013-2686-8

Interprofessional Education Collaborative. (2017). *Resources.* Retrieved from http://ipecollaborative.org/resources.html

Kitson, A., Harvey, G., & McCormack, B. (1998). Enabling the implementation of evidence based practice: a conceptual framework. *Quality in Health Care, 7,* 149–158. doi:10.1136/qshc.7.3.149.

Kitson, A. L., Rycroft-Malone, J., Harvey, G., McCormack, B., Seers, K., & Titchen, A. (2008). Evaluating the successful implementation of evidence into practice using the PARiHS framework: Theoretical and practical challenges. *Implementation Science: IS, 3*(1). doi:10.1186/1748-5908-3-1.

Luke, D. A., Baumann, A. A., Carothers, B. J., Landsverk, J., & Proctor, E. K. (2016). Forging a link between mentoring and collaboration: A new training model for implementation science. *Implementation Science, 11,* 137. https://doi.org/10.1186/s13012-016-0499-y

Morris, Z. S., Wooding, S., & Grant, J. (2011). The answer is 17 years, what is the question: Understanding time lags in translational research. *Journal of the Royal Society of Medicine, 104*(12), 510–520. https://doi.org/10.1258/jrsm.2011.110180

National Cancer Institute. (n.d.). *What is team science?* Retrieved from https://www.teamsciencetoolkit.cancer.gov/public/WhatisTS.aspx

National Center for Advancing Translational Sciences (NCATS). (2015a, March 12). *Translational science spectrum.* Retrieved from https://ncats.nih.gov/translation/spectrum

National Center for Advancing Translational Sciences (NCATS). (2015b, March 13). *About the CTSA Program.* Retrieved from https://ncats.nih.gov/ctsa/about

National Center for Advancing Translational Sciences (NCATS). (2015c, March 13). *CTSA program hubs.* Retrieved from https://ncats.nih.gov/ctsa/about/hubs

Patient-Centered Outcomes Research Institute. (2016, June 24). *Research infrastructure.* Retrieved from https://www.pcori.org/about-us/our-programs/research-infrastructure

Pinnock, H., Barwick, M., Carpenter, C. R., Eldridge, S., Grandes, G., Griffiths, C. J., . . . Taylor, S. J. C. (2017). Standards for Reporting Implementation Studies (StaRI) statement. *BMJ, 356,* i6795. https://doi.org/10.1136/bmj.i6795

Powell, B. J., Beidas, R. S., Lewis, C. C., Aarons, G. A., McMillen, J. C., Proctor, E. K., & Mandell, D. S. (2017). Methods to improve the selection and tailoring of implementation strategies. *The Journal of Behavioral Health Services & Research, 44*(2), 177–194. https://doi.org/10.1007/s11414-015-9475-6

Powell, B. J., Waltz, T. J., Chinman, M. J., Damschroder, L. J., Smith, J. L., Matthieu, M. M., Proctor, E. K., & Kirscher, J. (2015). A refined compilation of implementation strategies: Results from the Expert Recommendations for Implementing Change (ERIC) project. *Implementation Science. 10* (21) doi: 10.1186/s13012-015-0209-1 (pg. 9).

Rycroft-Malone, J. (2004). The PARIHS framework: A framework for guiding the implementation of evidence-based practice. *Journal of Nursing Care Quality, 19*(4), 297–304.

Straus, S. E., Tetroe, J., & Graham, I. (2009). Defining knowledge translation. *CMAJ: Canadian Medical Association Journal, 181*(3–4), 165–168. https://doi.org/10.1503/cmaj.081229

Wooten, K. C., Calhoun, W. J., Bhavnani, S., Rose, R. M., Ameredes, B., & Brasier, A. R. (2015). Evolution of multidisciplinary translational teams (MTTs): Insights for accelerating translational innovations. *CTS: Clinical & Translational Science, 8*(5), 542–552. https://doi.org/10.1111/cts.12266

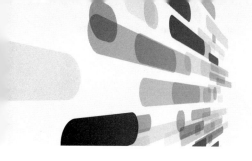

Case Exemplar

▶ Case Study 1

Collaboration and Implementation Science

Linda Roussel

Building on the concept of collaboration from an implementation science perspective has been the focused work of the Clinical Translational Science Awards (CTSA) hubs on a multi-site research platform perspective. The partner CTSA hubs became aware of the limited study on the implementation process, specifically noting the chasm between evidence generated and actions taken to implement evidence into routine clinical and public health practice (Kerner et al., 2005). Effective interventions "tested" under controlled research settings do little to illuminate the challenges and barriers to translating findings into real-world settings. Considering the translational perspective is essential to reaching the longer-term goal of improving research impact to the broader population, resulting in value-added returns on scientific investments. The National Implementation Research Network (NIRN, 2015) defines implementation science as the study of factors that impact the full and effective use of innovations in practice. The aim is not to answer factual questions about what is but rather to determine what is required to make the change or improvement. The National Institute of Health (NIH) has made implementation science (T3–T4 research) a priority, launching CTSAs in 2006. We have noted growth in implementation science, specifically moving from a set of studies chronicling the many barriers and facilitators to successful adoption, uptake, and sustainability. The past decade has experienced the movement toward comparing implementation strategies to implementation as a matter of course and more recently to the comparison of multiple active strategies (Proctor, Powell, & McMillen, 2013). In tandem, researchers have been advancing the methods and measures of implementation science by focusing on greater rigor and robustness of complex processes (Neta et al., 2015). With this backdrop, CTSA hubs have conceptually developed a platform using implementation science and collaboration to advance frontline engagement and nursing-sensitive outcomes. Through a robust virtual collaboratory, the CTSA hubs and their clinical teams would focus on sharing implementation strategies to improve key critical patient care and systems outcomes, such as reducing readmission rates, reducing length of stay, improving transitions of care, and reducing hospital-acquired conditions (HACs).

Reflection Questions

1. What is the process for building a virtual collaboratory from an implementation science perspective?
2. How may one address challenges associated with partner hubs within a virtual environment?

References

Kerner, J. F., Guirguis-Blake J., Hennessy, K. D., Brounstein, P. J., Vinson, C., Schwartz, R. H., et al. (2005). Translating research into improved outcomes in comprehensive cancer control. *Cancer Causes Control, 16*, 27–40.

National Implementation Research Network (NIRN). (2015). *Implementation science defined*. Retrieved from http://nirn.fpg.unc.edu/learn-implementation/implementation sciencedefined

Neta, G., Glasgow, R. E., Carpenter, C. R., Grimshaw, J. M., Rabin, B. A., Fernandez, M. E, et al. (2015). A framework for enhancing the value of research for dissemination and implementation. *American Journal of Public Health, 105*, 49–57.

Proctor, E. K., Powell, B. J., McMillen, J.C. (2013). Implementation strategies: Recommendations for specifying and reporting. *Implementation Science, 8*, 139.

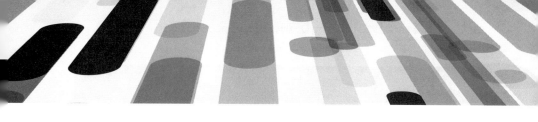

CHAPTER 4

Differentiating Quality Improvement Projects and Quality Improvement Research

Linda Roussel

ROLES

Advocate   Leader

PROFESSIONAL VALUES

Evidence-based practice   Quality
Patient-centered care

CORE COMPETENCIES

Assessment   Leadership
Coordination   Management
Design   Risk mitigation

▶ Introduction

The Health Resources and Services Administration (HRSA, 2011) defines **quality improvement** as a systematic and continuous process that leads to measurable improvement in healthcare services and the health status of a targeted patient population. As a process for improving quality outcomes, strategies are employed in an intentional way to assure that there is flow from the gaps (needs assessment) to the planning, implementing, and evaluation phases. The Institute of Medicine (IOM, 2001) defines quality in health care as a direct relationship between the level of improved health services and the expected health outcomes of individuals and populations. Quality improvement strategies are integral to projects that focus on safety, improvement, and **innovation**. Studying improvement interventions and possible research study types informs quality improvement research. Understanding the basic principles of quality improvement and quality improvement research is the cornerstone of projects that are impactful and add **value**.

This chapter seeks to define quality improvement and identify the primary elements in the quality improvement cycle. How quality improvement projects and quality improvement research are differentiated is described as well. In addition, this chapter considers related **improvement sciences**, such as translational and implementation science.

▶ Quality Improvement

Quality improvement requires thoughtful leadership in nursing as a major driver in advancing positive healthcare outcomes. Shewhart (1931) first studied quality from an industrial perspective, which led him to introduce concepts such as customer needs, reduction in variations in process, and elimination of the need for frequent inspections. Intrigued by Shewhart's work, Deming (1982) was able to determine that quality was a major driver for positive outcomes in industry; in turn, he introduced quality methodology to post-World War II Japanese engineers and executives. Deming's methods were strategically applied by the Japanese automobile industry, which enabled members of this industry—and other Japanese industries—to gain worldwide recognition for the quality of their products and services (Deming, 1982). Shewhart's and Deming's work on quality control has since informed the work of the Institute for Healthcare Improvement (IHI) and the Model for Improvement (MFI). The MFI is considered foundational to many of the quality models, such as Six Sigma, Lean Toyota, and the define–measure–analyze–improve–control (DMAIC) process (IHI, 2015a).

From the IOM's perspective, quality is considered within an organization's current system and is defined as how work gets done. Healthcare performance, however, is defined based on the organization's efficiency, care outcomes, and patient satisfaction levels. Quality is directly aligned with an organization's service delivery approach or underlying systems of care. Innovation is necessary to achieve a different level of performance and improve quality. From a **project planning** and management perspective on improving quality, it is important to understand the principles underpinning quality initiatives. The IOM purports that while a quality project may be unique to the organization, all successful quality initiatives integrate four key principles:

1. Quality improvement work as systems and processes
2. Focus on patients
3. Focus on being part of the team
4. Focus on use of the data

▶ Quality Improvement as Systems and Processes

If an organization is to make improvements, then understanding its own delivery system and key processes is critical to beginning this work. Quality improvement approaches recognize available resources (inputs) and tasks carried out (processes), which collectively determine quality of care (outputs/outcomes). For example, inputs may include people, infrastructure, materials, information, and technology. Consideration is given to the professionals and providers within the system, as well as to the supplies and equipment needed to carry out the project. According to Portela Pronovost, Woodcock, Carter, & Dixon-Woods, (2015), quality improvement projects tend to be applied, and in some cases, self-evaluating. While not directed at generating new knowledge, quality improvement projects may add considerable understanding of evidence-based uptake if the work is well conducted and cautious in their inferences (Portela et al. 2015).

Processes involve activities focusing on what is to be done and how the project will be carried out. Consequently, process-flow maps and concept maps are useful tools in illustrating the steps in carrying out the work. The process map, which comes to health care from engineering, provides a visual diagram that chronicles events or steps culminating in particular outcomes. The visualization of those steps provides a concrete look at how the work (process) is carried out, as well as who is accountable for that work and how efficiently the work flows, and can illuminate areas for improvement. Knowledge of how work flows may indicate the need for redesign, and the proposed plan can be compared to previous processes that are not working. In a blog post, IHI faculty members Little and Barbati (2015) describe five steps for creating value through process mapping and observations. The *first step*, identifying a care segment that has opportunities for improvement, involves looking at care segments with high consumption of resources, such as labor, supplies, time, and space. Opportunities for improvement could also include eliminating nonvalue-added clinical and administrative tasks. Interviewing experts (people involved in the process) and developing a first draft of a care segment process map is the *second important step* of process improvement. Preparing a list of frequently asked questions can be useful in optimizing the interviewee's time and talents. *Third,* it is best to start with Post-It notes, later converting to an electronic process map. This step allows for recognizing missing steps and illuminating misunderstandings, and it facilitates the ability to refer back to it for improvement opportunities. A *fourth step* involves observing the care segment twice to validate the process map. Repeating the process twice allows for "catching" variations and provides a perspective on the general flow of expectations that can be validated from the team's practice experiences. A *fifth step* includes connecting the dots (closing the loop) with practice experts after the observation experience. This involves sharing findings with subject-matter experts and managers to further validate opportunities for improvement. This step also allows for identifying nonvalue-added processes, which may in reality be barriers, leading these processes, to only be occurring 20–40% of the time. Tools and improvement strategies can be found at the IHI's website (Little & Barbati, 2015).

Gaps in the process can lead to further explorations, such as a thorough failure model effect analysis (FMEA). FMEA is a tool used for risk mitigation, which is essential to achieving safe, quality outcomes (IHI, 2015b). This type of analysis requires that each step (or process) be assessed for severity and frequency, with a hazard score being constructed to summarize these results. High hazard scores (8 or greater) alert the improvement team that emergent action is needed, particularly when the processes involve more than a single point, have few or no controls, and are not detectable (IHI, 2015c).

Outputs or outcomes may consider results or patterns such as health services delivered, changes in health behaviors and health status, and patient satisfaction. Health service delivery systems may be small, simple, and straightforward, such as a well-baby clinic, or multilayered and complex, such as a large corporate proprietary system. The efficiency and efficacy of the system depend on the services being individualized and attending to specific needs within the system. When the system considers the resources, activities, and results that exist and that are desired, quality improvement projects and programs can be customized to address unmet needs.

▶ Focus on Patients

Patient-centered care is not a new concept; indeed, it has been reinforced as a competency for educating healthcare professionals in the 21st century (IOM, 2001). Patient-centered care evolved with resurgence of the holistic roots of health care and initially had limited appeal given the complexity of the present healthcare system. Defined as engaging patients in a true partnership, patient-centered care involves personalizing care to include patients' normal routines and values. Such aims were considered daunting objectives when first introduced, and unrealistic at best. With increased technology and patient involvement, however, the creation of a healing physical environment, including one in which spiritual and emotional needs are met, has become mainstream practice.

So important is patient-centered care that the Hospital Consumer Assessment of Healthcare Providers and Systems (HCAHPS) created a patient survey that affords patients the opportunity to share information about their experiences with the healthcare system. In other words, this standardized tool assesses the way care is provided from the patients' perspective. Considering care from the patients' perspective takes into account more than just clinical treatment, medications, and technology. While core measures provide data that evaluate hospitals' care quality, at a minimum from a standard-of-care perspective, the patient experience is not necessarily taken into consideration when evaluating overall care delivery. HCAHPS considers aspects of the healthcare experience that patients report are important to them on a personal level, such as communication with nurses and physicians, cleanliness and noise levels, pain control, and quality of discharge instructions and medication information. Publicly reported scores of individual hospital systems have health systems on high alert, given that patients can now compare the way care is delivered by various systems and decide which is the best fit for them as individuals. With the advent of value-based purchasing, HCAHPS data have become increasingly important as a basis for reimbursement, further informing and advancing patient-centered care. Responding to these demands by delivering patient-centered care has also become an important business imperative.

The healthcare system's focus on patients is an important measure of quality that considers the patients' needs and expectations. When a focus on patients is present, services are created and designed by paying attention to the following factors: systems that affect patient access; care provision that is evidence-based; patient safety; support for patient engagement; coordination of care with other parts of the larger healthcare system; and cultural competence, including assessing the health literacy of patients, patient-centered communication, and linguistically appropriate care (HRSA, 2011).

▶ Focus on Being Part of the Team

Quality improvement (QI) is a "team sport." QI as a team process denotes the importance of the team coming together to take advantage of the knowledge, skills, experience, and perspectives of individual providers and professionals within the team to make sustainable improvements and produce innovations. Team effectiveness can happen when the following elements are in play: considering the process or system as complex; acknowledging that no one person in an organization knows all the dimensions of an issue; recognizing that the process involves more than one discipline or work area; advocating for solutions that require creativity; and realizing that staff commitment and buy-in are needed.

Vickberg and Christfort (2017) describe four styles that give leaders and teams a common language for understanding how people work and focus on improving collaboration and interprofessional competency. According to the authors, the styles bring useful perspectives and unique approaches to making decisions, generating ideas, and addressing problems. Being able to identify styles provides a common nomenclature, allowing for team structures that can maximize diversity and inclusion. The four styles include *Pioneers, Guardians, Drivers*, and *Integrators*. The *Pioneers* are bold thinkers, creative, value risk, and trust their gut. They are imaginative, ignite energy, and focus on the big picture. *Guardians* appreciate order, rigor, and organizational stability. They are data-driven and want facts, figures, and research-driven evidence to support their decisions. They are pragmatic and are reluctant to take on risks, always weighing all sides of an argument before taking a thoughtful position. Valuing challenges, generating momentum, and getting results are characteristics of *Drivers*. That is, "drivers tend to view issues as black-and-white and tackle problems head on, armed with logic and data" (Vickberg & Christfort, 2017, p. 52). The fourth style, *Integrators*, value bringing teams together and making connections. Integrators are diplomatic, focused on gaining consensus, and believe that most issues are relative. They appreciate that relationships and responsibility to the team are of the utmost importance. Intuitively bringing these styles together in teams could be beneficial for cognitive diversity, increasing creativity and innovation, and improving decision-making. In the authors' research, most top leaders are Pioneers or Drivers and report concern for groupthink due to their vocal styles. Guardians and Integrators were noted as being more stressed-out than any other styles; thus, looking for ways to maximize their strengths and easing their stress by making them feel psychologically safe are essential strategies for maximizing team effectiveness (Vickberg & Christfort, 2017).

Vickberg and Christfort (2017) provide strategies for managing the styles, specifically, pulling opposites closer, elevating the "tokens" on the team, and paying close attention to sensitive introverts (p. 54). Pulling opposites closer together can be accomplished by starting on small projects, then taking on bigger ones as the team opposites create complementary partnerships on the team. By generating productive friction and appreciating the differences, leaders can facilitate powerful collaborations. Elevating minority styles can enhance team functioning. For example, if you are trying to elicit Guardians' perspective, it is best to give them time and the details they need to prepare for a discussion or a decision, allowing them to contribute in ways that are comfortable for them, for example, in writing. This allows them the opportunity to have their "voice heard" without having to compete for the floor because they likely will not push to speak. Pioneers' ideas are often expansive, so providing whiteboards and encouraging others to use the markers available for interacting through sharing ideas would be important to increasing contributions and collaboration. Planning timed discussions ahead of the meetings will allow Guardians, who prefer structure, the opportunity to relax into the free-flowing exercise. Vickberg and Christfort recommend that the team leader ask members to brainstorm ahead of the scheduled meeting so that the roundtable discussions may be conducted in a way that allows the team leader to give the floor to members who may be reticent to offer their ideas. A useful strategy if there are few members of a particular style is to ask team members to "think like" that style and doing so early on in the meeting so that the majority viewpoint does not dominate the discussion (p. 55). Paying close attention to sensitive introverts involves encouraging anyone in the minority to share their "voice" early on, before dominant styles forge ahead. Guardians and quiet integrators often are risk aversive and so will see no reason to render their opinion to challenge prevailing wisdom. Team leaders who fail to recognize the various styles (particularly the quiet Integrators and Guardians) may miss the benefits of these styles. For example, these styles tend to be conscientious, thorough, and good at spotting errors and potential risks as they can focus intensely for long periods of time. Because they are good listeners, these styles often highlight others' great ideas and often take on and excel at the detail-oriented work that Pioneers and Drivers may prefer to pass on. While it may seem labor intensive to "draw out" these quieter styles by slowing the pace, reducing information overload, providing quieter and more private work environments, or running interference so that they can focus with minimal distractions, the benefits outweigh the costs.

All QI projects engage individuals as part of a team and implement QI as a team process. Projects such as improving time to referring providers, increasing patient engagement, reducing wait time, and ensuring providers' use of evidence-based guidelines are team efforts that can go far toward achieving sustainable improvements. Active involvement of team members is critical, as each individual skill set and contribution leads to a synthesis and synergy of ideas and solutions that would not have the same impact if they were implemented in isolation.

Another key component of a well-organized and functioning QI team is an effective infrastructure, such as leadership and policies/procedures that design and facilitate the work of the team. A strong infrastructure provides the team with tools, resources, clarity of expectations, and a medium for communication (HRSA, 2011).

▶ Focus on the Use of Data

A centerpiece of QI is the use of data. Data can be used to determine how effectively current systems are working and what occurs when changes are applied, and to document successful performance. By using data, the team is able to accomplish a number of tasks. First, the QI team members are able to separate what they believe is happening from what is actually happening within the system. A baseline can then be established to determine which, if any, changes made would be an improvement. It is likely that baseline scores will be low (this is acceptable), so the aim is to improve the rates and scores (e.g., patient satisfaction, falls, pressure ulcers, wait times, restraint use). By tracking data and comparing the baseline to the post-intervention data, the team can determine the efficacy of solutions; likewise, by monitoring procedural changes, it can evaluate whether improvements are sustained over time. In this way, data serve as powerful sources by which to determine whether the changes made led to improvements, and they allow for comparisons of performance across sites.

Quantitative and qualitative methods of collecting data are essential to QI projects. The use of numbers (rates, scores) and frequencies represents a quantitative research method that results in measurable data. Statistical process control, for instance, provides a wealth of information that can measure efficiency in care delivery. Examples include calculating how frequently patients access the emergency room and receive adequate health screenings. While numbers, rates, and frequency provide excellent ways to measure improvement efforts, the use of qualitative methods sheds light on the depth and breadth of the experience of care delivery. Data that are qualitative in nature are observable (not measurable), consider patterns and relationships between systems, and are contextual in nature. Qualitative methods may include patient and staff satisfaction surveys, focus groups, interviews, and participant-observation experiences.

Healthcare organizations can obtain data from a number of sources, including health records, patient and staff satisfaction surveys, external evaluations from accrediting and regulatory agencies, and community assessments. Using data sources in a methodical way within the infrastructure of an organizational system illuminates opportunities for improvement and allows for ongoing monitoring. Standardized performance measures focus on specific data for QI programs. Healthcare organizations are encouraged to collect data on performance measures that are impactful and add value to both the patient experience and the overall operation of the healthcare system. Such outcomes should guide the organization's decisions regarding which data are collected and measured.

▶ Quality Improvement Programs and Quality Improvement Research

With a QI program, the QI team considers the systematic activities that are designed and implemented to monitor, assess, and improve the organization's quality of health care for the population it serves. Higher levels of performance are reflected upon when reviewing the cyclical activities that are implemented to optimize resources and services for the patients served. There is a creative tension between innovation, sustained improvement, and ongoing delivery of evidence-based standards of care. Organizational QI programs incorporate all QI activities within the healthcare system.

The Donabedian model of structure, process, and outcomes provides a theoretical framework for integrating quality improvement strategies within the system (Donabedian, 1988). Leadership and interdisciplinary teams are essential to sustained quality improvement programs. Likewise, knowledge of the infrastructure and the principles of quality improvement is foundational to a successful QI program. Leaders ask the question of how QI processes work to support the success of the QI program. A number of benefits can be achieved from implementing a QI program, including improved patient (clinical) outcomes that focus on process outcomes (screenings) and health outcomes (blood glucose and blood pressure readings within normal parameters). Other benefits of QI programs are improved efficiency of managerial and clinical processes, such as reducing waste and maintaining financial viability.

According to HRSA, by improving processes and outcomes that reflect high-priority health needs, a system is able to reduce costs associated with system failures and redundancy. QI processes are typically budget-neutral, meaning that the costs incurred to make the changes are offset by the savings obtained through those efforts. QI programs put proactive processes in place and solve problems before they occur, making sure that systems of care are consistent, reliable, and predictable. These actions can go far in creating a culture of improvement, as they ensure that errors are tracked, reported, and addressed. Critical issues are often resolved because greater attention is paid to monitoring improvement initiatives and variations in standards of care.

Portela et al. (2015) offer ways to study improvement interventions using a variety of study types. The authors' literature search included reviewing a number of institutional sites, including *The Health Foundation, Institute for Healthcare Improvement, and Improvement Science Research Network*. Principles, strengths, weaknesses, and opportunities for study designs for improvement interventions are described. For example, considering quality improvement projects, the authors found that quality improvement projects should incorporate a theoretical base and qualitative methods in a more systematic way to allow for predicting and explaining the mechanisms for change involved. The authors note that more scientific rigor is needed in the application and reporting of Plan-Do-Study-Act (PDSA) cycles and other methods/techniques applied. Effectiveness studies, including randomized controlled trials (RCTs), quasi-experimental designs, observational (longitudinal) studies, and systematic reviews, are described. Specifically, strengths of systematic reviews are their ability to generate more powerful evidence, while weaknesses include uncritical incorporation and interpretation of studies, leading to inadequate conclusions. Low use of meta-analyses was also noted. The authors go on to report that due to the growth of systematic reviews on the effectiveness of quality improvement interventions, there is a need for more critical appraisal of the studies, including more meta-analyses, and to deal with complex interventions in diverse contexts.

With a culture of improvement in place, communication is enhanced both within the system and among community organizations. Improved communication focused on quality may result in stronger clinical partnerships and open up funding opportunities. An effective QI program can result in a balance of quality, efficiency, and profitability in its achievement of organizational goals (HRSA, 2011).

▶ Quality Improvement Research

QI projects may come under the federal definition of research and may require institutional review board (IRB) review and approval if they involve human participants or individually identifiable data. QI programs and QI research should not pose any risk to individuals, infringe on individual privacy, or breach individual confidentiality. Research in this context is defined as follows: 45 CFR 46.102(d) of the federal regulations defines research as a systematic investigation, including research development, testing, and evaluation designed to develop or contribute to generalizable knowledge (Reproduced from the *Institutional Review Board Guidebook* (1993). http://www.hhs.gov/ohrp/archive/irb/irb_chapter1.htm. Accessed February 8, 2015.)

One characteristic that distinguishes a QI program from QI research is whether the activities are intended or created to develop or contribute to generalizable knowledge. Results or research findings, when they are generalizable knowledge, can be applied to populations or situations beyond those being immediately studied. When quality improvement initiatives are not intended to yield generalizable knowledge, IRB review is not mandatory.

In contrast, QI research that is planned in advance to go beyond the scope of the unit, department, or services would require IRB approval. For example, the QI team may want the results from its analysis and the interpretation of its quality initiative to be disseminated across a larger scope and to a broader community of scholars. In other cases, quality improvement research may be intended for application beyond the current quality control efforts or improvements, as when new procedures or processes are shared with a larger audience (outside of one system).

If at least one of these descriptions of QI research applies to the team's QI plan, the next consideration would be whether the proposed activities and strategies are a systematic investigation. When applying the concept of systematic investigation, the team would determine whether information beyond what is routine for patient care will be collected. For example, adding surveys or more data collection through qualitative means, which is typically not part of routine care delivery, would go beyond a QI program. Another consideration with a systematic investigation would be to determine if the team will be assessing the effectiveness of processes or procedures and comparing two or more treatments, interventions, or processes. When such comparison is contemplated, and manipulation is done to determine if one practice is better, the effort would qualify as QI research. When QI activities entail a systematic investigation that will develop or contribute to generalizable knowledge, per 45 CFR 46.102(d), IRB review is mandatory (HHS, nd.).

QI research may be required for writing implementation research grants. Proctor, Powell, Baumann, Hamilton, and Santens (2012) provide 10 key ingredients, possibly best practices, for writing implementation research grant proposals. These ingredients include key questions to ask as well as review criteria. The 10 ingredients are as follows:

1. The care gap or quality gap
2. The evidence-based treatment to be implemented
3. Conceptual model and theoretical justification
4. Stakeholder priorities, engagement in change
5. Settings' readiness to adopt new services/treatments/programs
6. Implementation strategies/process
7. Team experience with the setting, treatment, implementation process
8. Feasibility of proposed research design and methods
9. Measurement and analysis section
10. Policy/funding environments, leverage or support for sustaining change (p. 3)

Taking into account the 10 key ingredients can strengthen your grant proposal. Review criteria are also offered and include significance impact, significance innovation, approach innovation, impact innovation, and environment. Knowing and responding to key questions and review criteria can best prepare the implementation science researcher in developing a strong, comprehensive grant proposal.

Specifically, when considering the implementation strategy/process ingredient, the researchers ask, "Are the strategies to implement the intervention clearly defined and justified conceptually?" The review criteria would include significance impact and innovation. Considering the ingredient of measurement and analysis section, the researcher would pose the following questions:

1. Does the proposal clarify the key constructs to be measured, corresponding to the overarching conceptual model or theory?
2. Is a measurement plan clear for each construct?
3. Does the analysis section demonstrate how relationships between constructs will be tested?

The review criteria to consider when focused on the measurement and analysis section takes into account the approach investigator team and provides key ways to address how the researchers will tackle this critical ingredient (Proctor et al., 2012).

At the outset, many QI projects have only local (organizational) assurance/improvement intentions; during the process of data collection or analysis, however, it may become clear that the findings could be generalizable or benefit others. In such a case, IRB review should occur—that is, IRB review is necessary whenever there is an intention to make findings generalizable.

▶ Quality Improvement and Beyond

While nurses are the largest subgroup in the healthcare system, they lack representation on decision-making bodies. QI activities can increase nurses' influence and involvement in decision-making at the policy level. A Gallup survey conducted by the

Robert Wood Johnson Foundation, titled "Nursing Leadership from the Bedside to the Boardroom: Opinion Leaders' Perception" (Gallup/Robert Wood Johnson Foundation, 2010), reported that the persons surveyed considered government executives (75%) and health insurance executives (56%) as being able to exert more influence on health reform than nurses, whom they ranked as having only 14% influence (Khoury, Blizzard, Moore, & Hassmiller, 2011). These numbers demonstrate that nurses, especially those in positions of authority, need to encourage the development of leaders within the profession and advocate for interprofessional QI team activity. Quality improvement programs provide an excellent opportunity for nurses to become involved in sustainable changes and policy development.

Beyond QI's immediate impact and results, consideration should be given to dissemination of both QI projects and QI research. Translational science, including improvement and implementation sciences, is also important to developing QI science.

Healthcare providers and consumers of health care are becoming more aware that research results that may have broad application do not always readily translate into improved health outcomes. The implementation and dissemination of research and science rely on a multidisciplinary set of theories and methods aimed at improving this process of translation from research evidence to pragmatic health-related practices. Implementation research, in particular, investigates how interventions can best be integrated into diverse practice settings and underscores direct engagement with the institutions and communities where health interventions are introduced. Team science and organizational and cultural perspectives are also integrated into translational science, as the gold standard of research (randomized controlled trials) often does not take into account the details necessary for application of findings.

Disseminating QI projects and research can take many forms, such as local stakeholder engagement; poster and podium presentations at regional, national, and international venues; and publication of manuscripts that share findings obtained, barriers overcome, and lessons learned. An excellent resource for dissemination of results is the Agency for Healthcare Research and Quality's (AHRQ) Health Care Innovations Exchange (AHRQ, n.d.). The Innovation Exchange is a web-based resource created to assist healthcare professionals in sharing and adopting innovations that improve healthcare quality. The website includes a clearinghouse of innovative ideas and opportunities to learn and share ideas with others.

Using research evidence to develop evidence-based practice guidelines is also important in the application and translation process of QI projects and research. The National Guidelines Clearinghouse (NGC) is another initiative of the AHRQ. It was originally created by AHRQ in partnership with the American Medical Association and the American Association of Health Plans (now America's Health Insurance Plans [AHIP]). The mission of the NGC is "to provide health professionals, healthcare providers, health plans, integrated delivery systems, purchasers, and others with a readily usable mechanism for accessing objective, detailed information on clinical practice guidelines and to further their dissemination, implementation, and use" (NGC, 2017).

QI projects and research can also be disseminated through manuscript submissions. A useful tool in writing up QI projects is the Standards for Quality Improvement Reporting Excellence (SQUIRE) guidelines. According to its sponsoring organization, the SQUIRE guidelines assist authors in writing up excellent, usable articles about quality improvement in health care. The guidelines serve as a way to report findings that may be easily discovered and widely disseminated. The SQUIRE website notes that high-quality writing about improvement, lists of available resources, and discussions about the writing process can enhance dissemination and adoption of best practices. Sponsors of the SQUIRE guidelines include the Dartmouth Institute for Health Policy and Clinical Practice, the Robert Wood Johnson Foundation, Quality and Safety in Healthcare, and the Institute for Healthcare Improvement (SQUIRE, 2017).

QI projects and research can also be shared through the Honor Society of Nursing, Sigma Theta Tau International. Its e-Repository hosts communities and collections that can be accessed and applied in practice, as well as a method of disseminating quality projects and research. According to the website, the Henderson Repository, a resource of Sigma Theta Tau International, offers the following benefits:

- *Online dissemination.* This global digital service collects, preserves, and shares nursing research and evidence-based practice materials.
- *Free open access.* There is no charge to submitting nurse authors and no access fee for online patrons.
- *Peer review.* Submissions to collections under the Independent Submissions community are peer reviewed. (Sigma Theta Tau International, n.d.)

Dissemination of evidence and information takes many forms, and methods for quality improvement and quality improvement research can be shared with many colleagues through these means. Evidence-based journal clubs and clinical scholars' programs are other ways to raise the level of conversation, create a spirit of inquiry, and enhance the culture of improvement in health care.

▶ Summary

- Quality improvement projects and quality improvement research share common aims for making healthcare systems safe and quality-driven.
- Leading a quality team that is focused on patient-centered care and using data to inform the process are essential to the work of clinical nurse leaders, executive leadership students, doctors of nursing practice (DNP), and highly functioning interprofessional project teams.
- The foundational work for the development of quality improvement projects and research is key to sustaining success over the long term.

Reflection Questions

1. Describe quality improvement projects you are currently involved in as part of your practice immersion experience.
2. Using the styles described by Vickberg and Christfort (2017), identify the styles in your team meeting, outlining strategies in place to increase team members' contributions and collaboration.
3. Access the AHRB Innovation Exchange, and select an innovation that best aligns with your quality improvement work. How are you able to use the evidence and strategies described for the innovation?
4. Access the National Guideline Clearinghouse (NGC). Which guideline can you adopt in providing evidence-based care to your own patient populations?

References

Agency for Healthcare for Research and Quality. (n.d.). *Innovation Exchange*. Retrieved from https://innovations.ahrq.gov

Deming, E. W. (1982). *Out of crisis*. Cambridge, MA: MIT Center for Advanced Engineering Study.

Donabedian, A. (1988). The quality of care: How can it be assessed? *Journal of the American Medical Association, 260*(12), 1743–1748. doi:10.1001/jama.1988.03410120089033

Gallup/Robert Wood Johnson Foundation. (2010). *Nursing leadership from bedside to boardroom: Opinion leaders' perceptions*. Retrieved from http://www.rwjf.org/content/dam/web-assets/2010/01/nursing-leadership-from-bedside-to-boardroom

Health and Human Services (HHS). (n.d.). *Office of Human Research Protections. Federal policy for the protection of human subjects* ("common rule"). Retrieved from https://www.hhs.gov/ohrp/regulations-and-policy/regulations/common-rule/index.html

Health Resources and Services Administration (HRSA). (2011). *Quality improvement*. Retrieved from http://www.hrsa.gov/quality/toolbox/methodology/qualityimprovement

Institute for Healthcare Improvement (IHI). (2015a). *The breakthrough series: IHI's collaborative model for achieving breakthrough improvement*. Retrieved from http://www.ihi.org/resources/Pages/IHIWhitePapers/TheBreakthroughSeriesIHIsCollaborativeModelforAchievingBreakthroughImprovement.aspx

Institute for Healthcare Improvement (IHI). (2015b). *Failure mode effect analysis tool*. Retrieved from http://www.ihi.org/resources/Pages/Tools/FailureModesandEffectsAnalysisTool.aspx

Institute for Healthcare Improvement (IHI). (2015c). *How to improve*. Retrieved from http://www.ihi.org/resources/Pages/HowtoImprove/default.aspx

Institute of Medicine (IOM). Committee on Quality Health Care in America. (2001). *Crossing the quality chasm: A new health system for the 21st century*. Washington, DC: National Academy Press. Retrieved from http://www.iom.edu/About IOM.aspx

Khoury, C. M., Blizzard, R., Moore, L. W., & Hassmiller, S. (2011). Nursing leadership from bedside to boardroom: A Gallup national survey of opinion leaders. *Journal of Nursing Administration, 41*(7/8), 299–305.

Little, K., & Barbati, M. (2015). 5 steps for creating value through process mapping and observations. *Institute of Healthcare Improvement [Blog post]*. Retrieved from http://www.ihi.org/communities/blogs/5-steps-for-creating-value-through-process-mapping-and-observation

National Guideline Clearinghouse (NGC). (2017). *Help & about*. Retrieved from https://www.guideline.gov/

Portela, M. C., Pronovost, P. J., Woodcock, T., Carter, P., & Dixon-Woods, M. (2015). How to study improvement interventions: A brief overview of possible study types. *BMJ Quality & Safety, 24*, 325–336. doi:10.1136/bmjqs-2014-003620

Proctor, E. K., Powell, B. J., Powell, A., Baumann, A. A., Hamilton, A. M., & Santens, R. L. (2012). Writing implementation research grant proposals: Ten key ingredients. *Implementation Science, 7*(96). Retrieved from http://www.implementationscience.com/content/7/1/96

Shewhart, W. A. (1931). *Economic control of quality of manufactured product*. New York, NY: D. Van Nostrand.

Sigma Theta Tau International. (n.d.). *Virginia Henderson Global Nursing e-Repository*. Retrieved from http://www.nursinglibrary.org/vhl

Standards for Quality Improvement Reporting Excellence (SQUIRE). (2017). *Revised standards for quality improvement reporting excellence SQUIRE 2.0*. Retrieved from http://squire-statement.org

U.S. Department of Health and Human Services (DHHS). (1993). *Institutional review board guidebook*. Retrieved from https://www.hhs.gov/ohrp/education-and-outreach/archived-materials/index.html

Vickberg, S. M. J., & Christfort, K. (2017, March–April). Pioneers, drivers, integrators, and guardians. *Harvard Business Review*, 50–57.

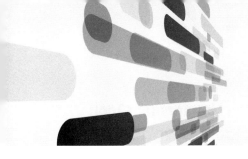

Case Exemplars

▶ ## Case Study 1

Quality Teams Approach to Discharge Planning

Terri Poe

A team of doctor of nursing practice (DNP) students engaged their quality team at their practice site to improve discharge planning by reducing nonvalue-added activities. The students, working together as a team of acute care nurse practitioners (ACNPs), noted a pattern of increasingly long waits for patients to be transferred to another level of care. To confirm that the pattern they experienced was a "true gap," they engaged their team members, the quality committee, and the chief nurse executive (CNE) to share their concerns. To obtain data to examine the outcomes, they were required to submit a question and begin a search of the external evidence. Through their translational courses, the students were able to step through the quality improvement process, beginning with obtaining internal data through a microsystems analysis and a failure mode effect analysis (FMEA), identifying a gap, searching for external evidence (synthesizing the research), and working with the Model for Improvement to begin a small test of change. As they progressed in their quality improvement work, they were able to bring team members along by charting a team, examining the process (through a process flow map), and using plan–do–study–act (PDSA) as a methodological framework for their scholarly project.

Reflection Questions

1. How can faculty best assure that doctoral students and interprofessional teams consistently go through a quality improvement process in which they will be able to engage their local stakeholders?
2. After completing the first iteration of the PDSA method, what would you suggest is the best way for doctoral students and teams to disseminate their results from the first cycle?

▶ Case Study 2

Action Plans as an Effective Asthma Management Tool: A Proposed Quality Improvement Project

Heather Surcouf

Asthma affects more than 22 million Americans. Asthma exacerbations lead to missed school, low quality of life, missed days on the job, hospitalizations, and emergency room visits. Multiple studies support asthma action plans (AAPs) as effective tools for asthma management.

At one school-based health center in Louisiana, the AAP completion rates declined markedly after adoption of an electronic health record (EHR). A project utilizing electronic health record reminders to prompt providers to complete AAPs was proposed. These reminders were set up to "pop up" in the EHR when an AAP is due. The provider recorded which action was taken (e.g., AAP completed, rescheduled, canceled) to move beyond the pop-up. These reminders automatically did the reset to appear on a yearly basis. The project relied on the Donabedian Model of Quality Care for theoretical structure. The Deming cycle and plan–do–study–act (PDSA) method of quality monitoring were used to assure continued quality improvements.

Specific project goals included the following: (1) increased provider AAP completion rates, (2) continued Office of Public Health clinic funding secondary to AAP benchmark satisfaction, and (3) reduced asthma exacerbation–related clinic visits. Congruent with the guidelines of the American Association of Colleges of Nursing (AACN), and advanced nursing practice (DNP Essentials), this project evaluated provider use of information systems and technology to support and improve patient care using the AAP (AACN, 2006, p.12).

Records of patients with asthma (ages 14–21) were audited both before and after project implementation for the presence of a completed, up-to-date AAP. Pre-implementation data and post-implementation data for two separate 9-month periods were compiled through a retrospective review of the electronic records of patients seen in the clinic for a 9-month period prior to the study and for a 9-month period after the study's implementation, based on their diagnosis of asthma. Records included for review were determined through the electronic record's reporting program. Results were tabulated using a frequency table (i.e., the number of patients with asthma with a completed AAP and the number of patients with asthma without a completed AAP). A second frequency table was used to tally the number of asthma-related visits for the same study periods using identical ICD-9 codes. Lastly, providers were given an anonymous survey before and after the intervention to gauge their familiarity with EHR reminders as well as their opinion regarding their effectiveness.

Reflection Questions

1. What is the value of an action plan in managing clinical symptoms?
2. How can medical record reminders promote patient-centered care delivery?
3. Identify tools that are useful in implementing quality improvement projects. Which of the tools are most useful when developing and implementing projects?

References

American Association of Colleges of Nursing (AACN). (2006). *Doctor of nursing practice (DNP) essentials.* Retrieved from http://www.aacnnursing.org/Education-Resources/AACN-Essentials

Bibliography

Bell, L. M., Grundmeier, R., Localio, R., Zorc, J., Fiks, A. G., Zhang, X., . . . Guevara, J. P. (2010). Electronic health record-based decision supports to improve asthma care: A cluster-randomized trial. *Pediatrics, 125*(4), e770–e774. doi:10.1542/peds.2009-1385

Centers for Disease Control and Prevention. (2007, May 4). *CDC vital signs: Asthma in the U.S.* Retrieved from http://www.cdc.gov/vitalsigns/asthma

Ducharme, F. M., & Bhogal, S. K. (2008). The role of written action plans in childhood asthma. *Current Opinion in Allergy and Clinical Immunology, 8*(2), 177–188. Retrieved from http://www.ncbi.nlm .nih.gov/pmc/articles/PMC3522127

Halterman, J. S., Fisher, S., Conn, K. S., Fagnano, M., Lynch, K., Marky, A., & Szilagyi, P. G. (2006). Improved preventive care for asthma: A randomized trial of clinician prompting in pediatric offices. *Archives of Pediatrics and Adolescent Medicine, 160,* 1018–1025. Retrieved from http:// archpedi.jamanetwork.com; links.com/index.php

Tolomeo, C., Shiffman, R., & Bazzy-Asaad, A. (2008). Electronic medical records in a sub-specialty practice: One asthma center's experience. *Journal of Asthma, 45*(9), 849–851. doi:10.1080/02770900802380803

Turkelson, C., & Hughes, J. E. (2006). Why aren't you doing evidence based practice? [Reprint]. *AAOS Bulletin, 54*(3), 1–4. Retrieved from http://www5.aaos.org/oko/ebp/EBP001/suppPDFs /OKO_EBP001_S23.pdf

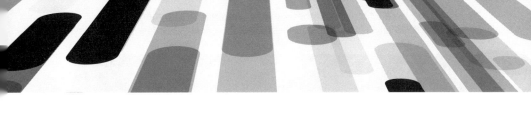

CHAPTER 5

Literature Synthesis and Organizational Alignment to Project Interventions and Implementation

Catherine Dearman
Lolita Chappel-Aiken
Katrina Davis

CHAPTER OBJECTIVES

1. Examine the process for synthesizing literature findings to form the basis for project development and dissemination.
2. Design a matrix to facilitate a synthesis of literature and evidence.
3. Use the synthesis matrix to align the literature and evidence with project objectives to create a seamless transition.

KEY TERMS

Evidence
Organization and Alignment

Project Interventions
Synthesis Matrix

ROLES

Faculty	Manager
Leader	Reviewer

PROFESSIONAL VALUES

Quality	Synthesis, Writing, and Organization
Evidence Evaluation and Grading	

CORE COMPETENCIES

Analysis	Design
Synthesis	Development
Alignment	

▶ Introduction

Synthesizing and organizing relevant literature that is aligned or can be aligned to your project objectives and implementation plan is an essential component of translating evidence into practice and designing quality improvement projects. Synthesis is defined as "the composition or combination of parts or elements so as to form a whole" (Synthesis, n.d.). Ultimately, the result of synthesis is the development of a new, higher level of knowledge regarding a subject of interest. The compelling attributes of synthesis are that it involves higher-order thinking skills and focuses on the production of something new and unique—something that has not occurred before—like your project.

Individuals synthesize information on a daily basis. New parents review multiple daycare agencies, synthesize the evidence, and choose the best one for them and their child. Students synthesize information from peers and relevant sources to determine which professor's course they will take. Busy mothers synthesize information about their work schedule and their children's activities so that they can assure they have constructed an appropriate plan of attack.

The skill of synthesis thinking and writing is essential to the development of new ideas and forms the basis of quality improvement projects such as those conducted by doctor of nursing practice (DNP), clinical nurse leader (CNL), and nurse executive students. Synthesis thinking and writing seeks to address a gap in evidence or clinical practice (Hain & Kear, 2015). You may not have developed your synthesis writing skill set yet; however, it is integral to your combination of critical thinking and creative reasoning in the development of a unique project. In the following pages, the aspects of analyzing and categorizing evidence into relevant structures; the synthesis of available evidence into new, unique projects; and the **alignment** of the evidence to your project objectives/implementation plan will be discussed in detail. Such evidence includes "best research evidence, clinical expertise, and values of the patient or subject" (Roberts, 2013, p. 5). Finally, tools, guidelines, and techniques for categorizing and synthesizing evidence that aligns with your project will be presented.

▶ Literature Synthesis and Best Available Evidence

The primary aspect of literature synthesis begins with the supporting evidence. Writers must search for and critically appraise all available evidence in order to clearly identify what is known and not known about the topic, to establish a reliable knowledge base, and to highlight opportunities for the new project (Briner & Denyer, 2012). According to Glasgow, Green, Taylor, and Stange (2012), "translation of . . . evidence to . . . practice has been conceptualized as a linear process—a pipeline or roadmap which is slow and inconsistent" (p. 646). These authors propose a different way to conceptualize translation processes, an evidence integration triangle to align science with practice. Similarly, Kilbourne, Neumann, Pincus, Bauer, and Stall (2007) proposed a replicating-effective-programs framework to facilitate the implementation of evidence-based interventions proposed through research or quality improvement projects. All of these mechanisms were predicated on effective collection and critical appraisal of the evidence.

A clear, comprehensive review of the literature is based on synthesis writing. Drew University has an online resource for writers regarding synthesis writing and describes the process as "combining two or more summaries in a meaningful way" (Drew University. n.d.) that supports the writer's thesis. Synthesis involves integrating themes or ideas from the literature into your thinking/writing and allows you to create a new, unique outcome. Synthesis is dependent on analysis of concepts, classifications, and categorizations but does not stop there. Synthesis involves the "search for links between materials for the purpose of constructing a thesis or theory" (Drew University, n.d.). which brings the disparate ideas and concepts into harmony, creating a meaningful new structure.

Synthesis writing can be achieved using an "explanatory" or an "argumentative" approach (Kelly, 2017). In the explanatory synthesis option, the writer is simply describing objectively without presenting a position or opinion. Argumentative synthesis writing involves the writer selecting a position and providing justification for that position. The argumentative option is more suitable for quality improvement or innovation projects because they require the writer to propose a new idea that is supported by existing literature but does not duplicate that literature. The idea is new and unique but is well founded in current evidence (Drew University, n.d.).

In either type of synthesis writing, the writer first proposes a one-sentence thesis statement, not a question, that will be the focus of the project (Drew University, n.d.). The thesis statement reflects the synthesis of supporting literature while identifying the innovation or improvement. The remainder of the paper is composed of paragraphs that provide detail from the literature and other evidence to help the reader see the information in a new way. Each paragraph reflects a blending of reference material, not a summary of each source, and is linked to one or more key elements or subtopics associated with the idea or project. The paper ends with a conclusion that addresses the "so what" and links back to the thesis (Kelly, 2017).

Synthesis writing is accurate, organized, and helps the reader make sense of information so that they can clearly see the overlaps and gaps in the available data. Again, to accomplish these aspects of synthesis writing, the writer must locate all studies, positive, negative, supportive, and contradictory, creating a clear path forward that is fully supported by existing evidence (Briner & Denyer, 2012). The paragraphs in a synthesized document are organized by topic or subtopic rather than by source and present a coherent assessment of the subject. Synthesis writing answers the question "what do we know about . . . (*the topic*)? The ultimate goal is to demonstrate that the writer is highly knowledgeable about the topic, has developed a perspective and/or interpretation of the evidence, and can assert that "no one has addressed XX," which will, in turn, become writer's project.

▶ Organization of Evidence

The guiding principle in organizing evidence is to lead the reader to the fact that your project is the only logical conclusion to the problem. Several tools and teaching methods exist in the literature that propose strategies for synthesis writing. Synthesize eLecture, Lippincott's Nursing Center.com, as well as several university writing centers provide writing advice and tools to help writers organize and effectively present evidence.

Most of the articles and websites propose beginning with a thesis statement worded similarly to this example: This project is going to address (*topic/issue/problem*) through (*strategy*). Writers can use this basic template and fill in the blanks with specifics related to their project.

Developing outlines is an effective way of organizing thoughts and events and will serve as an effective guide to writing the literature review. Some outlines are chronological; however, in the case of synthesis writing, the outline is based on the primary topics associated with the project or idea being proposed. Outlines may be more effective after content is organized using a synthesis matrix such as the one proposed in the Tools, Guidelines, and Techniques for Literature Synthesis and Project Alignment section later in the chapter.

▶ Aligning Evidence with Project Interventions and Implementation

Aligning supporting evidence with project interventions and implementation requires that the writer be very knowledgeable regarding the subject matter and all aspects of the project. The writer should locate all available resources, published and unpublished, that are linked to the project ideas and appraise the quality and relevance of the evidence to inform the project (Gough, 2007). The intent is to clearly establish that the writer is fully conversant with what is known and not known about the topic. Therefore, even negative and contradictory evidence must be unearthed and reviewed carefully. The writer should assure that all information in the review of the literature is supported by existing evidence. Evidence is broader than research findings alone and encompasses current clinical practices, the strategies that have worked in the individual agency or institution in prior projects, and even the writer's personal experiences (Glasgow et al., 2012). Ultimately, the object of aligning the existing evidence to the project objectives and implementation plan is to clearly highlight a "gap" in the knowledge base, which presents an opportunity for the project being proposed (Briner & Denyer, 2012).

Synthesis involves putting together ideas into a new or unique product or plan that presents a solution to a previously unanswered problem (Kelly, 2017). Glasgow et al. (2012) promote the use of a "straightforward and systematic" path from new idea to integration into practice (p. 646). Typical action verbs associated with synthesis thinking include create new ideas; predict, modify, or change a mechanism; and organize, adapt, elaborate, and draw conclusions regarding a topic or set of topics.

▶ Tools, Guidelines, and Techniques for Literature Synthesis and Project Alignment

Cognitive Maps

According to wisegeek.com, cognitive mapping is the "means through which people process with environment, solve problems and use memory." While cognitive maps are generally used to help learners connect new information to that previously learned, they can also be useful for writers trying to express a disparate data set. Synthesis writing uses topics and subtopics to organize a literature review. The cognitive map shown below (**FIGURE 5-1**) can also be used to diagram topics and subtopics prior to writing about them.

Synthesis Matrix

TABLE 5-1, adapted from a chart created by the North Carolina State University Writing and Speaking Tutorial Service (2006) (https://tutorial.dasa.ncsu.edu/wp-content/uploads/sites/29/2015/06/synthesis-matrix.pdf), provides a tabular view of the same information. To use the chart, enter comprehensive information as you review each article/reference. Once all the references are entered into the chart, you can develop an outline or write directly from the chart.

As you work through all the evidence you have collected, you may need to modify the matrix. Once the matrix is complete, it will serve to guide writing. As you enter the information into the matrix, you will begin to see how the data relate, or not. Not all sources will have information that fits into the matrix completely. Some may

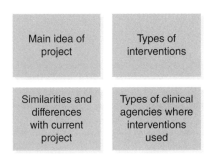

FIGURE 5-1 Cognitive Map

TABLE 5-1 Synthesis Matrix for Literature Review					
Author/ Title	Purpose of Project	Framework	Similarities/ Controversies to Your Project	Results	Implications for Practice, Research, and Theory

have more information; some may have less. If your completed matrix has gaps or areas where little or no information is included, these areas may guide your thinking about what is known and what is not known about the topic. Patterns of information may become readily visible within the matrix. All of this information will guide your synthesis of the evidence.

▶ Summary

- This chapter discusses a literature synthesis, methods of organizing the evidence, purposeful synthesis writing, and aligning evidence with the project interventions and implementation.
- Tools, guidelines, and techniques to assist the writer are provided to give a new perspective and interpretation of the evidence surrounding the project.

Reflection Questions

1. Why is it essential for the writer to identify, read, and synthesize data that both support and do not support the project?
2. What action verbs associated with synthesis writing provide the writer with a way to design an appropriate quality improvement project?
3. How is synthesis writing different from other types of writing? How does that difference impact aligning the evidence with project interventions and implementations?

References

Briner, R. B., & Denyer, D. (2012). Systematic review and evidence synthesis as a practice and scholarship tool. In D. M. Rousseau (Ed.), *Handbook of evidence based management: companies, classrooms and research* (pp.112-119). New York, NY: Oxford University Press.

Drew University. (n.d.). *Synthesis writing.* Retrieved from https://users.drew.edu/sjamieso/Webresources .html

Glasgow, R. E., Green, L. W., Taylor, M. V., & Stange, K. C. (2012). An evidence integration triangle for aligning science with policy and practice. *American Journal of Preventive Medicine, 42*(6), 646–654.

Gough, D. (2007). Weight of evidence: A framework for the appraisal of the quality and relevance of evidence. *Research Papers in Education, 22*(2), 213–228.

Hain, D. J., & Kear, T. M. (2015). Using evidence-based practice to move beyond doing things the way we have always done them. *Nephrology Nursing Journal, 42*(1), 11–21. Retrieved from http://152.12.30.4:2048/login?url=https://search.proquest.com/docview/1655480007?accountid=15070

Kelly, M. (2017). *Higher level thinking: Synthesis in Bloom's taxonomy: Putting the parts together to create new meaning.* Retrieved from http://www1.center.k12.mo.us/edtech/Blooms /Synthesis.htm

Kilbourne, A. M., Neumann, M. S., Pincus, H. A., Bauer, M. S., & Stall, R. (2007). Implementing evidence-based interventions in healthcare: Application of the replicating effective programs framework. *Implementation Science, 2*(42). https://doi.org/10.1186/1748-5908-2-42

North Carolina State University. North Carolina State University Writing and Speaking Tutorial Service. (2006). *Writing a literature review and using a synthesis matrix.* Retrieved from https:// tutorial.dasa.ncsu.edu/wp-content/uploads/sites/29/2015/06/synthesis-matrix.pdf

Roberts, B. (2013). Doctor of nursing practice: Integrating theory, research, and evidence-based practice. *Clinical Scholars Review, 6*(1), 4–8. Retrieved from http://152.12.30.4:2048/login?url=https://search .proquest.com/docview/1348259634?accountid=15070

Synthesis. (n.d.) In *Merriam-Webster's online dictionary.* Retrieved from https://www.merriam-webster .com/dictionary/synthesis?src=search-dict-box

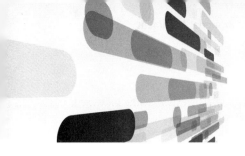

Case Exemplars

▶ Case Study 1

Synthesis Writing (Hand Hygiene)

The DNP student has identified a rise in hospital-acquired infections that is limited to the medicalsurgical units. Hand-hygiene protocols are in place on all units throughout the facility. The DNP student wishes to compare the protocol to actual practice and identify a gap for project development. The first step is to identify and synthesize the literature and evidence from practice.

Sample of Synthesis Writing Related to Hand Hygiene

Hand hygiene is one of the most effective methods for preventing infection (Aziz, 2013; Mortell, 2012; Spruce, 2013). In the mid-1800s, Dr. Semmelweis was one of the first physicians to recognize the importance of hand hygiene for preventing infection (Aziz, 2013; Molinari, 2017; Mortell, 2012). There is a lack of adherence to hand-hygiene protocols among healthcare workers (Aziz, 2013; Mortell, 2012). This can lead to an increase in healthcare-associated infections, spreading drug-resistant micro-organisms (Molinari, 2017; Mortell, 2012). Some reasons for nonadherence to hand hygiene include a lack of priority, allergy to or intolerance of antiseptics, and a lack of leadership (Mortell, 2012; Spruce, 2013). It is important to increase hand-hygiene compliance because it can improve patient outcomes (Molinari, 2017; Mortell, 2012).

Identification of Gap

The standard hand-hygiene protocols currently in place need to be assessed to determine compliance and to improve health outcomes.

Thesis Statement for Project Development

This project will compare current standard hand hygiene protocol to clinical practice on three specific medical surgical units to determine compliance.

References

Aziz, A. (2013). How better availability of materials improved hand-hygiene compliance. *British Journal of Nursing*, *22*(8), 458–463.

Molinari, J. A. (2017). Effective, sensible, and safe hand hygiene: Poor compliance among clinicians still leads to associated infections. *RDH*, *37*(10), 62–65.

Mortell, M. (2012). Hand hygiene compliance: Is there a theory-practice-ethics gap? *British Journal of Nursing*, *21*(17), 1011–1014.

Spruce, L. (2013). Back to basics: Hand hygiene and surgical hand antisepsis. *AORN Journal*, *98*(5), 449–460. doi:10.1016/j.aorn.2013.08.017

▶ Case Study 2

A community-based, nurse-led, family-centered practice is experiencing increased numbers of patients exhibiting hypertensive issues. The vulnerable, low-income, and predominately African American patient population has been provided with literature on best practices with regard to management of hypertension. Nutritionists have provided evidence-based meal plans for each of the patients. Pharmacological treatments have been prescribed for all.

Yet, the majority of patients are not experiencing a decrease in their blood pressure. The Clinical Nurse Leader student is interested in this issue and has devised a protocol to identify causes, relational factors, and patient views as a basis for a clinical innovation project.

Reflection Questions

1. What process should she follow?
2. What literature does she need to review?
3. What practice policies does she need to review?
4. What practice standards exist that may or may not be being used in this practice?
5. What steps does the CNL student need to take to assure comprehensiveness of the project?

CHAPTER 6

The Institutional Review Board Process

Catherine Dearman
Dionne Roberts
Lolita Chappel-Aiken

CHAPTER OBJECTIVES

1. Examine the process for initiating and completing the institutional review board (IRB) process—the when, why, and how to navigate the process.
2. Formulate a crosswalk that features the parts associated with initiating and completing the IRB process.

KEY TERMS

Human-subject protection
Human subjects

Informed consent
Institutional review board (IRB)

ROLES

Participant
Researcher

Reviewer

PROFESSIONAL VALUES

Beneficence   Respect for persons
Quality   Social justice

CORE COMPETENCIES

Analysis   Design
Communication   Development

▶ Introduction

This chapter reviews the role of the **institutional review board (IRB)** in an organization and describes the basic process used in the review of a study. The institutional review board is integral to the protection of **human subjects** and connecting those subjects to the protocols and safeguards included in completing an IRB application. Organizations sponsoring research and other scholarly work must consider the impact of that work on human subjects and be able to determine whether information gleaned from the work can be generalized to the public. Therefore, IRB approval should be secured prior to any data collection for research and quality improvement projects.

The IRB comprises a representative group of faculty and staff within an institution who are experienced in research processes and thoroughly understand how the rights of subjects in the research are protected. The IRB reviews all research and many quality improvement protocols involving human subjects prior to their implementation, to assure that subjects' human rights are protected. In many cases, IRB approval is a basic requirement to publication of the findings, including those from quality improvement projects.

Inherent in the IRB review is the independent nature of the review and the reviewers—that is, researchers do not review their own work, but rather, independent members of the IRB review each submission. In some cases, more than one IRB will need to be involved in the review of the research, especially if the university is not connected to the clinical facility where the research will occur.

Regardless of the project that is identified, the initial step is to complete a needs assessment, analyze the data, and assimilate data as background support when building the business case. However, one cannot dismiss the need to obtain IRB approval if the data or outcomes of a project will be disseminated beyond the immediate organization or system. Securing IRB approval at the beginning of the project limits future issues.

▶ Historical Perspective Related to Protection of Human Subjects

The Federal Policy for the Protection of Human Subjects requires universities or other institutions that receive federal funds and conduct biomedical or behavioral research involving human subjects to establish an institutional review process.

The "Common Rule," as the policy is widely known, requires a research institution to assure the protection of the human rights of human subjects who participate in research. The institution is bound by law, then, to assure that all researchers follow this rule with regard to selecting subjects and obtaining **informed consent** from them (U.S. Department of Health and Human Services, [DHHS] 2011, 2012).

IRBs emerged based on principles included in the Nuremberg Code (U.S. GPO, 1949), the Declaration of Helsinki (World Medical Association, 2008), and the Belmont Report (National Commission for the Protection of Human Subjects of Biomedical and Behavioral Research, 1979). These documents define the minimum codes for conducting research with human beings, as well the ethical principles of beneficence, respect, and justice, which form the basis for all human research endeavors. The concept of beneficence assures that the study is structured in such a way that it will benefit—and not harm—the subjects. Researchers must then address the risks and benefits inherent in the research for all participants. Respect for persons and their right to choose to participate or not, as well as their right to cease participation at any point, is addressed through the informed consent process. Justice addresses the potential for all persons to be included in the study; no single person or group—and particularly not a vulnerable person or group—can be singled out to receive benefits or harm from the research (National Commission for the Protection of Human Subjects of Biomedical and Behavioral Research, 1979).

What is a human subject? Human subjects are living participants who are working with one or more researchers who are studying a phenomenon to acquire data by involvement (can be via distance; not required to be face-to-face) or data that can be used to distinguish one phenomenon from another.

▶ The History of the Human-Subjects Protection System

Human-subject protection began with the Nuremberg Code, which was developed for the Nuremberg Military Tribunal as a standard against which to judge the human experimentation conducted by the Nazis during World War II. The Nuremberg Code captures many of what are now taken to be the basic principles governing the ethical conduct of research involving human subjects. Its first provision states that "the voluntary consent of the human subject is absolutely essential" (U.S. GPO, 1949). Freely given consent to participate in research is the cornerstone of ethical experimentation involving human subjects. The Nuremberg Code also provides the details implied by such a requirement—namely, capacity to consent, freedom from coercion, and comprehension of the risks and benefits involved. Other provisions require that risk and harm be minimized, that the risk/benefit ratio be determined and shared with the potential subjects of the research, that qualified investigators use appropriate research designs, and that subjects have the freedom to withdraw at any time.

Similar recommendations were made by the World Medical Association in its *Declaration of Helsinki: Recommendations Guiding Medical Doctors in Biomedical Research Involving Human Subjects*, first adopted by the 18th World Medical Assembly in Helsinki, Finland, in 1964 and subsequently revised by the 29th World Medical Assembly, Tokyo, Japan, 1975, and by the 41st World Medical Assembly, Hong Kong, 1989 (World Medical Association, 2008). The Declaration of Helsinki further distinguishes therapeutic from nontherapeutic research (Steneck, 2007).

In the United States, regulations protecting human subjects first became effective on May 30, 1974. These regulations were promulgated by the Department of Health, Education and Welfare (DHEW) and raised to regulatory status in 1966 as the National Institutes of Health's (NIH) Policies for the Protection of Human Subjects. The regulations established the IRB as one mechanism through which human subjects could be protected.

In July 1974, the National Commission for the Protection of Human Subjects of Biomedical and Behavioral Research was established. The Commission met from 1974 to 1978 and issued reports identifying the basic ethical principles that should underlie the conduct of biomedical and behavioral research involving human subjects and recommending guidelines to ensure that research is conducted in accordance with those principles. Its report setting forth the basic ethical principles that should underlie the conduct of biomedical and behavioral research involving human subjects is titled *The Belmont Report: Ethical Principles and Guidelines for the Protection of Human Subjects of Research.* The Belmont Report, which is named after the Belmont Conference Center at the Smithsonian Institution, sets forth the basic ethical principles underlying the acceptable conduct of research involving human subjects. Those principles—respect for persons, beneficence, and justice—are now accepted as the three quintessential requirements for the ethical conduct of research involving human subjects and are discussed below:

- *Respect for persons* involves a researcher and his or her team recognizing the personal dignity and autonomy of individuals and providing for special protection of those persons with diminished autonomy.
- *Beneficence* entails an obligation to protect persons from harm by maximizing anticipated benefits and minimizing possible risks of harm.
- *Justice* requires that the benefits and burdens of research be distributed fairly (National Commission for the Protection of Human Subjects of Biomedical and Behavioral Research, 1979).

The Belmont Report also describes how these principles apply to the conduct of research. Specifically, the principle of respect for persons underlies the need to obtain informed consent, the principle of beneficence underlies the need to engage in a risk/benefit analysis and to minimize risks, and the principle of justice requires that subjects be fairly selected. As was mandated by the congressional charge to the National Commission, the Belmont Report also provides a distinction between "practice" and "research." The text of the Belmont Report is thus divided into two sections: (1) boundaries between practice and research, and (2) basic ethical principles (DHHS, 2010a).

The DHHS regulations are codified at Title 45 Part 46 of the Code of Federal Regulations and became final on January 16, 1981; these regulations were revised effective March 4, 1983, and June 18, 1991. The 1991 revision involved the adoption of the Federal Policy for the Protection of Human Subjects. The Federal Policy ("Common Rule") was promulgated by the 16 federal agencies that conduct, support, or otherwise regulate human-subjects research; the Food and Drug Administration (FDA) also adopted certain provisions. The Federal Policy is designed to make the human-subjects protection system uniform in all relevant federal agencies and departments. Additional protections for various vulnerable populations have been adopted by the DHHS reflecting vulnerable populations such as pregnant women (August 8, 1975; revised January 11, 1978, and November 3, 1978), prisoners (November 16, 1978), and children (March 8, 1983, and revised June 18, 1991) (DHHS, 2010a).

An account of the history of human-subjects research and the human-subjects protection system in the United States can be found in Rothman's *Strangers at the Bedside: A History of How Law and Bioethics Transformed Medical Decision Making* and in Maloney's *Protection of Human Research Subjects*. Rothman details the abuses to which human subjects were exposed, culminating in Beecher's 1966 article, "Ethics and Clinical Research," published in the *New England Journal of Medicine*, and ultimately contributing to the impetus for the first NIH and FDA regulations (Fain, 2009).

▶ Definition of Research

Research is a "diligent and systematic inquiry or investigation into a subject in order to discover or revise facts, theories, applications . . ." (Research, n.d.). The intent to publish findings is generally considered as contributing to generalizable knowledge. An investigation, then, must meet certain criteria to be classified as research. Research studies are designed in an organized, logical process that can support a range of goals, from basic scientific inquiry to a qualitative research study of a specified group. Research processes, measurement, assessment, and data collection are required elements of the study itself. Essentially, research is completed in a manner that will allow findings, experiences, or understandings gleaned from the work to be generalized to the broader population. Some research involves rodents, larger animals, or even primates. These studies are evaluated differently than research involving human subjects. When humans are involved, the research processes and procedures that include consent forms and the issue of informed consent must be evaluated by an IRB (DHHS, 2010b).

The research project is usually described in a formal protocol that sets forth an objective and a set of procedures designed to reach that objective. The Belmont Report recognizes that "experimental" procedures do not necessarily constitute research, and that research and practice may occur simultaneously. It suggests that the safety and effectiveness of such "experimental" procedures should be investigated early, and that institutional oversight mechanisms, such as medical practice committees, can ensure that this need is met by requiring that "major innovation[s] be incorporated into a formal research project" (National Commission for the Protection of Human Subjects of Biomedical and Behavioral Research, 1979).

▶ Boundaries Between Practice and Research

Why discuss IRBs when quality improvement processes and quality assessments are the foci for most clinical nurse leaders (CNLs), nurse executives, doctor of nursing practice (DNP) candidates, and other clinical doctorate students? If the IRB is predominantly focused on the ethical conduct of research, then why should quality improvement projects be reviewed by the IRB? After all, quality improvement is not research, is it? While recognizing that the distinction between research and therapy is often blurred, practice is described as interventions that are designed solely to enhance the well-being of an individual patient or client and that have a reasonable expectation of success. The purpose of medical or behavioral practice, then, is to provide diagnosis, preventive treatment, or therapy to particular individuals.

Ultimately, patients are the focus of quality improvement/process improvement projects, and their rights must be protected (Speers, 2008); the IRB process offers that protection. Similarly, community needs assessments can impact individuals and populations; thus, their protection is also warranted.

Quality improvement activities are widely regarded as critical to the effort to reduce healthcare errors and improve patient outcomes. Most can be readily distinguished from research; however, some cannot (Speers, 2008). The issue for students in nurse executive, clinical nurse leader, and DNP programs is that they are not generating new knowledge; instead, they are testing and offering translation of research findings into practice and the care of patients. To share with colleagues a project's success in improving quality of care, results are published, which brings quality improvement projects into the realm of research.

In 2007, national attention was brought to the impact of quality improvement studies on patient care. In turn, many healthcare professionals became involved in heated arguments about the differences between research and quality improvement. For example, a major care provider implemented a checklist for insertion of large intravenous (IV) lines in patients. As a part of this checklist, providers were reminded to wash their hands prior to the procedure and to wear sterile gloves and a gown. Within 3 months, IV line infection rates fell precipitously, resulting in a simultaneous reduction in costs for the provider. However, because the checklist was determined to be an intervention that impacted patients and no consent had been obtained from those patients, the Office of Human Research Protection closed down the program. This was done despite the benign nature of the intervention and the significantly positive outcomes realized for patients.

As a result of these events, more attention is now being paid to process and quality improvement projects and drives the review of projects by IRBs. The problem that most students and project managers face with regard to completion of the application to the IRB for projects is that the application uses research language, not quality improvement language. Students frequently attempt, in error, to reconcile quality improvement projects with research language, such as describing an experimental design when presenting an intervention.

The information that IRB members need with regard to quality improvement projects is generally confined to the "W" questions and answers: What will be done? Who will do it, and Who will be involved in it? When will it be done (include stages)? Where will it be done, and how will it impact processes in the location(s)? Why is it necessary (include the potential impact on practice and improving health care)? In addition to these questions, the researcher/project manager needs to answer the "How" questions: How will the project unfold? How long will it take? How will the impact be measured? Clarity is essential in the application process; students and faculty should seek help on an as-needed basis.

▶ Applying the Ethical Principles to Both Research and Quality Improvement

The responsible conduct of research (RCR) requires investigators involved in any level of the research to complete basic training in the protection of human subjects. Scholarship in the health sciences requires a clear understanding of the ethics involved in conducting research. This basic training can be obtained through the National Institutes of Health (NIH) or the Collaborative Institutional Training Initiative (CITI) modules (CITI, 2011; NIH, 2011).

Respect for Persons

RCR training addresses the ethical principles of respect for persons. Informed consent to participate in research or a quality improvement project is required by the ethical principle of "respect for persons." It includes three elements: information, comprehension, and voluntariness.

First, potential subjects must be given sufficient information to be able to decide whether to participate, including the research procedures, their purposes, risks and anticipated benefits, alternative procedures (where therapy is involved), and a statement offering the subject the opportunity to ask questions and to withdraw at any time from the research. Incomplete disclosure is justified only if it is clear that (1) the goals of the research cannot be accomplished if full disclosure is made; (2) the undisclosed risks are minimal; and (3) when appropriate, subjects will be debriefed and provided with the research results.

Second, subjects must be able to comprehend the information that is given to them. The presentation of information must be adapted to the subject's capacity to understand it; researchers may be required to test potential subjects to assure they understand. Where persons with limited ability to comprehend are involved, they should be given the opportunity to choose whether to participate (to the extent they are able to do so), and their objections should not be overridden. Each such class of persons should be considered on its own terms (e.g., minors, persons with impaired mental capacities, the terminally ill, and the comatose).

Third, consent to participate must be voluntarily given. The conditions under which an agreement to participate is made must be free from coercion and undue influence. IRBs are especially sensitive to these factors when particularly vulnerable subjects are involved.

Beneficence

The principle of beneficence addresses risk/benefit assessments and includes information on the probability and potential magnitude of possible harms and benefits. Researchers must define the nature and scope of the risks and benefits while systematically assessing them. All possible harms—not just physical or psychological pain or injury—should be considered. The principle of beneficence requires both protecting individual subjects against risk of harm and considering not only the benefits for the individual but also the societal benefits that might be gained from the research.

Justice

The principle of justice mandates that the process used to select research subjects must be fair and must result in fair selection outcomes. The "justness" of subject selection relates both to the subject as an individual and to the subject as a member of social, racial, sexual, or ethnic groups.

With respect to their status as individuals, researchers need to assure that certain persons (poor, racial or ethnic minorities, or those who are institutionalized) are not selected simply because they are available or their circumstances are easily manipulated (NIH, Office of Extramural Research, 2011).

▶ Informed Consent

The process of assuring that the participants in research or quality improvement projects are aware of their rights and the three primary principles of respect for persons, beneficence, and justice is termed *informed consent*. Informed consent documents must present the information clearly and in readily understandable language without esoteric terms or convoluted sentence structure or word use.

The two primary elements to be addressed in the informed consent process are the provision of complete information about the study/project and the understanding of the participant regarding that information. Providing information alone is not sufficient to meet the standard of informed consent—the participant must also fully understand what they he or she is agreeing to as a part of the study/project.

Some key elements of informed consent were discussed previously in relation to respect for persons, beneficence, and justice. However, some populations may be fully informed and voice understanding yet not truly understand. Such may be the case with individuals with low literacy, for example. Options for assisting those with low literacy skills include reading the consent form for the participant and allowing sufficient time for the participant to consult with another individual, such as a family member or clergy.

Another special case arises with children who participate in research/projects. Parents must provide consent for all minors participating in research. The children, too, must give permission (assent) to be involved in the study. In cases where higher risks are associated, the researcher may be required to obtain assent from the child as well as consent from both parents.

Typically, informed consent takes the form of a signed, written document. However, a waiver of written informed consent can be approved if the presence of a signed document could increase the risk associated with participation. It is significant to note that the waiver, if used, applies only to the signed written document; it does not apply to the actual process of informing the participants.

Informed consent is as essential in quality improvement projects as in research studies. Any participant in any organized project must be afforded his or her rights, including informed consent.

▶ Institutional Review Board Processes and Procedures

Having to complete an IRB application can appear to be quite complicated and off-putting, but the process actually is straightforward and procedurally oriented. When one considers that the overall purpose of the IRB is to protect human subjects, the process becomes fairly benign.

IRB reviewers look for clear explanations of what will be done, who will do it, when it will be done, and how it will be done so that the board members can determine if the project requires full board review or is eligible for expedited or exempt status. A clear understanding of the intent of the project is critical to the IRB review process. The discussion that follows highlights some ways to respond to the nature of the question without categorizing the quality improvement project in research terms while assuring ready understanding by IRB review teams. Some of the areas of the application are readily discernable, and others take a bit more information.

The remainder of this section provides details on the information needed to complete an IRB application. The basic processes the application will follow during the staged review are also addressed.

Research Purpose

Typically, the researcher needs to provide a brief description of the intent of the project. This section is basically the same for research studies or quality improvement projects. The applicant needs to answer the question: What is the problem, and which impacts will the proposed research/project have?

Subject or Population

Who will be involved in the project and how? To which population will the results be generalizable? Again, this section is the same for research studies or for quality improvement projects, even though findings from quality improvement studies are not typically considered to be generalizable to larger populations due to agency variations. Basically, the information presented must allow investigators, institutions, or IRBs to determine if the proposed methods of selecting participants could result in unjust distributions of the burdens and benefits of research. For example, subjects should not be selected simply because they are readily available in settings where research is conducted or because they are "easy to manipulate as a result of their illness or socioeconomic condition" (DHHS, 1993).

Design of the Study

This section is very different for research studies and quality improvement projects. The applicant will need to provide enough information for reviewers to determine if the design fits the purpose and has the potential to yield the anticipated outcomes.

For research studies, the discussion of study design should address the overall nature of the study—experimental, quasi-experimental, descriptive, or mixed methods. Applicants must provide specific aims that the research will address and explain how the design will facilitate achieving those aims. Some indication of the underlying quantitative or qualitative focus is included.

For quality improvement (QI) studies, the QI design must be linked to the project and to the project site as well as to the quantitative and/or qualitative nature of the project. Some typical QI designs are the FADE model (focus, analyze, develop, and execute), PDSA (plan–do–study–act), and Six Sigma. Six Sigma actually encompasses two different models: DMAIC (define–measure–analyze–improve–control) and

DMADV (define–measure–analyze–design–verify), which are used for existing and new processes, respectively. The basic premise is the same regardless of which design is specified: Reviewers must know how the project will be conducted.

Privacy and Confidentiality

How will the researcher protect the information collected? Will participants be recognizable? Will responses be linked to participants? How and where will the data be stored? Who will have access? This last issue is particularly relevant to staff or patient participants who may fear retribution if they answer questions truthfully. In QI projects, participant pools are typically smaller and site-specific. The researcher must carefully assure that the privacy of all participants is protected.

▶ Inclusion/Exclusion Criteria

How will the researcher determine the eligibility of participants? The applicant must describe the processes and procedures used in determining who is eligible to participate in the research/project versus who is not eligible. The researcher will also need to ensure that the issue of vulnerability is addressed. Frequently, quality improvement projects do not include children or other vulnerable populations, although that is not a hard-and-fast rule. Consequently, the researcher must describe inclusion and exclusion criteria comprehensively. If a population or subgroup is excluded for any reason, the application must clearly address those criteria. The researcher must be aware that the IRB application may require a stipulation whether or not any vulnerable population is included.

Risks and Benefits from Participation

Even if they are minimal, the researcher needs to address all risks and benefits to the participant, actual or potential, including physical and psychological risks and benefits, inconvenience, and loss of privacy. If subjects will be paid to participate in the research, the amount of payment and the restrictions on the payment need to be explained in detail. With regard to risks and benefits, more attention is generally paid to the risks than to the benefits. Therefore, the IRB members must independently assess the risk to the participants to determine if they agree with the risk assessment in the application. Additionally, the IRB must determine the type, probability, and extent of the risk as much as possible. It must determine if the researcher's estimates of harm or benefit to participants are reasonable, given the facts and results of other studies.

Five basic principles apply to risk/benefit assessment:

1. "Brutal or inhumane treatment of human subjects is never morally justified."
2. Risks should be minimized, including the avoidance of using human subjects if at all possible.
3. IRBs must be scrupulous in insisting on sufficient justification for research involving "significant risk of serious impairment" (direct benefit to the subject or "manifest voluntariness of the participation").
4. The appropriateness of involving vulnerable populations must be demonstrated.

5. The proposed informed consent process must thoroughly and completely disclose relevant risks and benefits (IRBNet, 2012).

If the researcher or project manager offers compensation to participants, the IRB must also be cognizant of the amount and impact of that compensation. Is the compensation commensurate with the participation? Could the amount of compensation affect an individual's participation to the extent that it affects the outcomes of the project/research?

Outcomes

The researcher must describe how the findings will be used. Are the findings sufficient to propose a change in policy or practice, or will more research be needed with different groups, under different circumstances, or some other criterion?

For QI projects, will the project potentially change practice? How might that change occur? Whom will the change affect?

Informed Consent Form

A copy of the informed consent document is included in the packet provided to the IRB so that an assessment can be made with regard to the accuracy of information shared with participants and the reading level required to ensure true understanding.

▶ Levels of Institutional Review Board Reviews

The IRB has the authority to approve or not approve research and/or QI projects (Fain, 2009). IRB reviews occur on three distinct levels depending on the degree to which the study is considered to constitute potential harm or violation of one or more ethical principles. Those three levels are full review, expedited, and exempt (Polit & Beck, 2012). An applicant can request a specific level of review, but the final decision regarding that level rests with the IRB staff and committee.

The full review process requires that a full IRB committee, including scientific, nonscientific, and community members, evaluate the study. All members of the IRB read, consider, and evaluate each study. Primary and secondary reviewers are stipulated to present the salient facts of the study to the full board, including all components of human-subject protection. The researcher maintains responsibility for the responsible conduct of research, even with a full board review. A full board review is typically reserved for studies with inherent risks to participants. Examples of studies that fit this criterion are those focused on sensitive topics such as race, ethnicity, and sexual behaviors; studies focused on vulnerable populations; and clinical trials, especially related to medication regimens.

Expedited reviews are reserved for studies in which "minimal" exposure to risk is projected. Minimal risk is defined as the participants being at no greater risk than they could encounter as a part of daily life. Expedited reviews are typically conducted by one or two members of the IRB committee and are reported at the IRB meeting but not discussed there. Many QI projects qualify for an expedited review, as they constitute minimal risk to subjects.

An exempt review designation is typically reserved for studies where no human subjects are involved or for studies where there is no risk to humans. Typically, exempt studies include situations where subjects cannot be identified, secondary review of existing data, studies in which data are gathered through observation of public behavior, and anonymous surveys (DHHS, 2010a).

▶ Multiple Institutional Review Boards

In most research studies, a single institutional review board is responsible for assuring compliance with human-subject protection. Typically, this review board exists within the primary agency/institution which maintains responsibility for the project. Once approval is obtained from this review board, evidence of that approval is provided to other partner agencies.

In the case of Quality Improvement projects, however, multiple IRBs may be indicated. The primary agency/institution's IRB is typically approached first. Clinical agencies where the project will be implemented may assert the need to file a separate application through their on-site IRB. This practice is becoming more commonplace as more clinical agencies have established IRBs.

▶ Summary

- This chapter has provided an overview of the role of the institutional review board (IRB) in an organization, a review of the basic processes involved in the review of a study, and methods involved in the protection of human subjects.
- The institutional review board is the primary mechanism used by institutions to ensure the protection of human subjects through informed consent, justice, beneficence, and respect for persons. The institutional review board also reviews quality improvement studies to ensure that human subjects are protected.
- Researchers must be aware of the institutional review board policies within their institutions and be prepared to complete the processes to ensure the protection of the persons involved in their research.

Reflection Questions

1. Which institutional criteria are used to review an IRB application?
2. What differentiates a quality improvement project from research?

References

Collaborative Institutional Training Initiative (CITI). (2011). *CITI course in the responsible conduct of research.* Retrieved from https://www.citiprogram.org/rcrpage.asp?language=english&affiliation=100

Fain, J. A. (2009). *Reading, understanding, and applying nursing research* (3rd ed.). Philadelphia, PA: F. A. Davis.

IRBNet. (2012). *Innovative solutions for compliance and research management.* Retrieved from https://www.irbnet.org

National Commission for the Protection of Human Subjects of Biomedical and Behavioral Research. (1979). *The Belmont report: Ethical principles and guidelines for the protection of human subjects of research*. Retrieved from http://www.fda.gov/ohrms/dockets/ac/05/briefing/2005-4178b_09_02 _Belmont%20Report.pdf

National Institutes of Health (NIH), Office of Extramural Research. (2011). *Protecting human research participants*. Retrieved from http://phrp.nihtraining.cm/users/login.php

Polit, D. F., & Beck, C. T. (2012). *Nursing research: Generating and assessing evidence for nursing practice* (9th ed.). Philadelphia, PA: Lippincott Williams & Wilkins.

Research. (n.d.). *Dictionary.com*. Retrieved from http://www.dictionary.reference.com/browse /research?s=t

Speers, M. A. (2008). Editorial: Quality improvement: Research or non-research? AAHRPP perspective. *Association for the Accreditation of Human Research Protection Programs, Advance, 5*(2), 1–2.

Steneck, N. H. (2007). *ORI: Introduction to responsible conduct of research*. Retrieved from https:// ori.hhs.gov/ori-introduction-responsible-conduct-research

U.S. Department of Health and Human Services (DHHS). (1993). *Institutional Review Board Guidebook*. Retrieved from https://www.hhs.gov/ohrp/education-and-outreach/archived-materials/index.html

U.S. Department of Health and Human Services (DHHS). (2010a). *Code of federal regulations*. Retrieved from http://www.hhs.gov/ohrp/humansubjects/guidance/45cfr46.html#46.html#46.102

U.S. Department of Health and Human Services (DHHS). (2010b). *Guidance on IRB continuing review of research*. Retrieved from http://www.hhs.gov/ohrp/policy/continuingreview2010.html

U.S. Department of Health and Human Services (DHHS). (2011). *Information related to advanced notice of proposed rulemaking (ANPRM) for revisions to the Common Rule*. Retrieved from https://www .hhs.gov/ohrp/regulations-and-policy/regulations/anprm-for-revision-to-common-rule/index.html

U.S. Department of Health & Human Services (DHHS). (2012). *The federal policy for human subject protections (The Common Rule)*. Retrieved from http://www.hhs.gov/ohrp/humansubjects /commonrule/index.html

U.S. Government Printing Office (GPO). (1949). *Trials of war criminals before the Nuremberg military tribunals under control council law 10*(2), 181–182. Retrieved from https://history.nih.gov/research /downloads/nuremberg.pdf

World Medical Association. (2008). *World Medical Association Declaration of Helsinki: Ethical principles for medical research involving human subjects*. Retrieved from https://www.wma.net/policies-post /wma-declaration-of-helsinki-ethical-principles-for-medical-research-involving-human-subjects

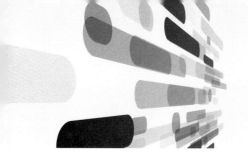

Case Exemplars

▶ Case Study 1

Vulnerable Population

Dionne Roberts

A doctor of nurse practice (DNP) student proposed a pediatric practice change to implement an intervention to increase the human papillomavirus (HPV) vaccination in the practice. The practice will discuss HPV prevention at each office visit, including sick visits. The intervention will involve the nursing staff, the preteen/adolescent patient, and a parent. The participant will be between 11 and 18 years of age. The DNP student will recruit at the practice for eligible participants. The nursing staff will let the DNP student know which patients meet the inclusion criteria and inform the patients that someone will come to discuss a potential study with them. In the recruitment session, it will require the DNP student to discuss a brief statement about the relationship of sexual activity and HPV with the possible participants. The preteen/adolescent and parent will both be in the session. The intervention will require the revision of the Centers for Disease Control and Prevention (CDC) HPV fact sheet to be discussed in 5 minutes with allocated time for questions. An HPV knowledge instrument will be used before and after the intervention.

Reflection Questions

1. With this type of DNP project, would this proposal require an expedited or full board review?
2. Would it be required for the preteen/adolescent to complete an assent form and the parent to complete an informed consent form?
3. Can the DNP student speak with the preteen/adolescent without the parent?

▶ Case Study 2

IRB Application for DNP Project

Dionne Roberts

With the DNP project proposal, there are sections that are included in the project that aren't commonly used with a research proposal. These sections will address topics such as the clinical mentor, stakeholders, resources, and quality improvement efforts. It can be challenging for the DNP student to change his or her DNP project proposal to an IRB application that has been geared toward a research project. The IRB application has a template that will highlight the sections and provide page limits. The DNP project's practice question stated as a PICOT (Population, Intervention, Comparison, Outcome, Time) question may be difficult for an IRB member who is not familiar with the practice-focused doctorate to understand. The research question guides the statistical analyses. If the research question is not stated accurately and clearly on the IRB application, it may be perceived that the statistical analyses may not be consistent with the research question. Review the IRB template—the DNP student may not need to submit the DNP information such as the SWOT (Strengths, Weaknesses, Opportunities, and Threats) analysis as part of the literature review. However, the methodology is important, and the DNP student needs to describe the quality improvement project in this section.

Reflection Questions

1. Has the PICOT question been changed to a similar research question?
2. Is the statistical analysis consistent with the research question?
3. Did you obtain a letter of support stating that you can conduct the DNP project at the appropriate clinic or practice?

▶ Case Study 3

The CNL Capstone Project: An Experiential and Transformative Process

Theodora Ledford

Differentiating quality projects from research often challenges students to ensure that the objective of the project is met and any impact on human-subjects' protection is determined. Upon completing a microsystem needs assessment and engaging in dialogue with the institutional review board, it was established that the clinical nurse leader (CNL) project was needed to obtain information that supported nursing quality improvement data. Data gleaned from the project would be useful for detecting trends in and patterns of performance that affected more than the identified microsystem. Data collected would be utilized in the development of action plans in collaboration with other practice committees concerning nurse-sensitive indicators directed at quality, safe, and efficient patient outcomes. Additionally, data could engender interprofessional collaboration, opportunities to monitor and evaluate compliance with standards, recommendations to enhance continuous quality improvements, and the spread of safety initiatives throughout the healthcare system.

While the capstone project started initially as an outcomes-based endeavor where differentiating quality improvement from research was of foremost importance, the transformative processes that followed were valuable. The experience culminated in thoughts of how unit-based quality nursing councils could use data to create more solid structures and processes. As a result, an innovative environment was envisioned where strong professional practice would flourish and the mission, vision, and values would come to life. This notion can become a reality. However, during dialogue with colleagues and quality improvement staff, a fundamental action was needed—namely, the development of a guide for other nurses to understand the differences between quality improvement projects and research and the steps necessary for accomplishing meaningful and value-added quality projects that are patient-centric and advance care delivery. Steps are in process for the action to become reality.

Reflection Questions

1. Which individual challenges do students confront when completing IRB applications for universities and clinical agencies?
2. How might students create opportunities from challenges associated with quality improvement and research endeavors?

CHAPTER 7

Synergistic Interprofessional Teams: Essential Drivers of Person-Centered Care

Patricia L. Thomas
Janet E. Winter

CHAPTER OBJECTIVES

1. Describe tools, strategies, and methods used to create synergistic interprofessional teams that are dedicated to effective project planning, management, and person-centered programs.
2. Discuss the importance of the stages of team development, synergy, transformational leadership, creativity, and innovation as interprofessional teams address outcomes through project/program management.
3. Assess the value and use of various metrics when evaluating interprofessional team effectiveness.

KEY TERMS

Ad hoc committee
Advocate
Appreciative inquiry
Brainstorming

Communicator
Decision-making
Group
Innovation

(continues)

KEY TERMS   (continued)

Interdisciplinary team
Interprofessional
Management
Multidisciplinary team
Program management
SBAR communication

Synergy
Task force
Team
TeamSTEPPS
Transdisciplinary team
Transformational leadership

ROLES

Advocate
Communicator
Decision maker
Integrator

Leader
Manager
Risk anticipation
Team member

PROFESSIONAL VALUES

Accountability
Altruism
Evidence-based practice

Integrity
Person/Patient-centered care
Quality

CORE COMPETENCIES

Appreciative inquiry
Assessment
Coordination
Critical thinking
Design

Interpersonal influence
Leadership
Management
Resource management
Systems thinking

▶ Introduction

Much has been written to stress the importance of **interprofessional** learning, the development of interprofessional **teams**, and the implementation of innovative interprofessional collaborative practices as new care delivery systems and practice settings evolve. While several distinct models have been developed to showcase changes needed in the practice and academic settings, implementation of these models and resultant sustained outcomes have been slow, sporadic, and inconsistent. Landmark reports from the Institute of Medicine (IOM) and the Robert Wood Johnson Foundation provide keen perspective by highlighting that while healthcare providers claim to value teamwork, communication, collaboration, and shared outcomes, they are plagued by professional assumptions, definitions, habitual use of language, and power structures.

In addition to dissonance around role and identity across various professions, the IOM's *To Err Is Human* report attributed preventable errors to organizational structures, incomplete information, failures in communication, and faulty systems and processes (IOM, 1999). Likewise, the IOM *Crossing the Quality Chasm* report emphasized that healthcare systems are not able to translate knowledge into practice related to quality and safety in large part because resources are not used effectively in fragmented systems where gaps and redundancies create waste and fail to achieve desired outcomes.

The Robert Wood Johnson Foundation and IOM published the *Future of Nursing: Leading Change, Advancing Health* (2010) report and made recommendations about how to transform the nursing workforce through education, leadership development and competencies, and use of data and information to address the gaps apparent in our current delivery systems. In light of these reports and recommendations, alignment and understanding of team dynamics, synergies that can be generated, and the need for creative and innovative models implemented by interprofessional teams is needed.

The six aims to improve patient care (safe, effective, patient-centered, timely, efficient, and equitable) are cornerstones to project **management** amid expectations for the delivery of cost-effective, high-quality care espoused in organizational mission, vision, and value statements. However, despite best efforts, these aims have not been accomplished consistently across the healthcare industry. Transformative change and investment in organizational capacity, building up of information infrastructure, and reconfiguration and retraining of care teams are needed (IOM, 2001).

Principles and constructs for teams and teamwork, team building, and team facilitation are extensive, spanning decades of work in nursing, business, and the social sciences. Recent alignment to safety, quality, and high-reliability organizations has catapulted the need for the implementation of effective team structure and processes through investment in project management team skills that ultimately drive optimum person-centered care.

Under the premise that project work can be accomplished through productive, high-functioning teams, this chapter will focus on key considerations in working with interprofessional as well as **interdisciplinary team** configurations during the project management processes of initiating, planning, executing, monitoring and controlling, and closing (Project Management Institute, 2013, p. 6).

Integral to this approach is an appreciation for current accomplishments, recognition of any voids or gaps, and an understanding of how new strategies and competencies should be leveraged to optimize team performance around project work.

▶ Types of Team Composition

Having an awareness of the different team member compositions can be helpful to consider when forming a team. Although terms are often used interchangeably, each composition offers nuances around member composition (see **TABLE 7-1**). For example, depending on the discipline or specialty, in healthcare literature there is a distinction between a **multidisciplinary team** and an interdisciplinary team. Interdisciplinary teams recognize the interdependence of members who come together to understand complex situations or solve complex problems that require the knowledge, skills, and abilities of diverse individuals who cannot be successful without one another. In this coming together of the individuals, recognition of overlapping roles is common, and

TABLE 7-1 Team Compositions	
Interdisciplinary	A group of healthcare professionals from diverse fields who work in a coordinated fashion toward a common goal for the patient.
Multidisciplinary	A team of professionals including representatives of different disciplines who coordinate the contributions of each profession, which are not considered to overlap, in order to improve patient care.
Intraprofessional	A team of professionals who are all from the same profession, such as three physical therapists collaborating on the same case.
Interprofessional	The inclusion of representatives from a particular discipline or knowledge branch with differing experiences, education, values, roles, and expectations (Zaccagnini & White, 2014).
Transdisciplinary/ Transprofessional	A team composed of members of a number of different professions cooperating across disciplines to improve patient care through practice or research.

unraveling the distinctions between them leads to an understanding of how each member's contributions could be woven together in a unique way to bring a new or different result. In contrast, multidisciplinary teams engage the knowledge, skills, and abilities of the members who work in parallel with distinct responsibilities to accomplish a shared goal. The former brings **synergy** and new possibilities, whereas the latter reinforces consistency in defined disciplinary outcomes (Nancarrow et al., 2013; Walters, 2012). However, while unique characteristics exist across team configurations, perhaps most importantly, each team composition connotes a purpose that aligns with any or all of the IOM's six aims.

In addition, team composition can promote unique interactions with regard to whether an individual's role interests or role knowledge support a team (interdisciplinary); when a professional's insights build from the conversations in a varied team (interprofessional); or when disciplines, professionals, and team members from seemingly unrelated fields come together to innovate to achieve a desired outcome (transdisciplinary or transprofessional) (Armstead, Bierman, Bradshaw, Martin, & Wright, 2016; Hewitt, Sims, & Harris, 2014; Mueller, 2016).

▶ Teams Versus Groups

Having a working knowledge of the differences between teams and **groups** is foundational to project or program success aimed at promoting person-centered care. Groups and teams hold attributes in common, but differentiation between attributes

TABLE 7-2 Interprofessional Teamwork versus Interprofessional Team-Based Care

Interprofessional Teamwork	The levels of cooperation, coordination, and collaboration characterizing the relationships between professions in delivering patient-centered care.
Interprofessional Team-Based Care	Care delivered by intentionally created, usually relatively small work groups in health care, who are recognized by others as well as by themselves as having a collective identity and shared responsibility for a patient or group of patients (e.g., rapid response team, palliative care team, primary care team, operating room team).

Reproduced from Interprofessional Education Collaborative. (2016). *Core competencies for interprofessional collaborative practice: 2016 update.* Washington, DC: Interprofessional Education Collaborative.

can sometimes explain why projects or programs derail. Groups and teams hold in common the gathering of individuals who come together to accomplish work. What distinguishes groups from teams is the degree of interdependence, how they are led, and who has ownership of the end product of the members' interactions. Groups have individual accountability to complete work, come together to share information, and complete individual work or tasks based on their role. The group members' purpose and goals are directed by a manager while they remain focused on their own challenges and interests. In contrast, teams have individual and mutual accountability; come together for discussion, problem solving, and planning; and collectively focus on achieving goals and outcomes. The team members' purpose, work, and goals are shaped by the leader with the members (Armstead et al., 2016; Braithewaite, 2015).

Analogies are often offered using sports examples to showcase the differences between groups and teams. With this being the case, marathon runners would serve as an example of a group. They have gathered for the same purpose, want to win, and share common interests. In terms of teams, thinking about baseball, soccer, or football teams, individual players come together but have to rely on each other to win. They have common goals but have to rely on the direction of the coach and the decisions and actions of their team members to ultimately achieve the "win." An individual could have a "great game" but still lose. For the purposes of project and **program management**, building teams rather than groups is the desired state.

Using a person-centered approach, the Interprofessional Education Collaborative (IPEC) Practice Competencies Panel (2011) distinguished teamwork from team-based care (**TABLE 7-2**).

▶ Individual Versus Team Performance

Determination about when the efforts of an individual versus the efforts of a team are needed is pivotal to success. There are times when individual choices, decisions, or actions enable success. Historically, the belief was held that individual actions, decisions, and accountability alone brought results. From this, silos of information and action were created, resulting in inconsistent and fragmented results, ineffective communication, and poor outcomes.

We have learned that success coming from collective efforts in complex systems rests in the ability to draw distinctions between when an individual's effort (commitment, participation, and actions) versus facilitated team efforts bring greater efficiency, effectiveness, and consistency aimed toward desired results. This tension between the individual team members' productivity and the team's overall productivity requires sensitivity among members on how their level of engagement affects the dynamics of the team in achieving desired goals. For example, timeliness in providing information integral to the workflow keeps the project moving forward, as does conveying only pertinent information needed for team **decision-making**. Conversely, an overabundance of extraneous information may overwhelm or distract team members, and inability to produce assigned work can contribute to delays in workflow.

As further expanded upon in the chapter, the role of the project manager or team leader involves systematically guiding the tension between individual and team productivity toward synergy over shared goals and shared language. In this, the unspoken assumption that goals and desired outcomes held by people in the same organization are the same because we care for the same patients and rely on a common mission and vision statement to guide our work is explored. To encourage team productivity, time is spent on setting team expectations and confirming the perceived meaning behind written, verbal, and nonverbal team member communications. This proactive approach clarifies and informs the use of communications that we may assume hold common meaning but in reality, due to education and experiences, have shaped our underlying assumptions in ways that are not consistent with others. Coming together over shared goals using shared language better positions a team to achieve successful outcomes integral to quality person-centered care.

▶ Team Structures

While the definitions for team configurations provide insight on member composition and focus, words used to describe the structure of teams provide perspective on the duration of work the team has been charged to accomplish. Committees, **task forces**, ad hoc teams, and councils represent common structures (and language) in healthcare organizations. Their permanency, charter, and purpose often determine how and why a team is established and guide the relevance attributed to organizational work. Committees and councils may result from expectations held by regulators (like The Joint Commission or state regulations) or governing boards and have defined responsibility and authority directed toward ongoing work. Task forces and ad hoc teams are often created to address an issue or need that has arisen. As such, their work is typically geared toward making recommendations aimed at an issue with the intent of informing leaders and disbanding (or transitioning into a newly created committee or council) (Danna, 2013; Walters, 2012).

▶ Stages of Team Development

Irrespective of team purpose, composition, or expected duration, there are stages of development that can be anticipated and observed in teams. The interactions between team members reflect the dynamic interplay between intrapersonal and interpersonal behaviors that contribute to the identity of the team. A commonly cited model in anticipating the evolutions within a team comes from the work of Bruce Tuckman (1965) and the revisions by Tuckman and Mary Ann Conover Jensen in 1977. The model is helpful in understanding team dynamics that begin with coming together and progress to find cohesiveness and synergy, produce outcomes, and then dissolve. The stages are also discussed in Chapter 8, as they are also relevant to managing interprofessional teams and their functions. The stages include the following:

Forming: Orientation where members define interpersonal boundaries and task behaviors.

Storming: Resisting group influence or task requirements, characterized by interpersonal conflict.

Norming: Resistance declines and cohesion emerges as expectations and roles are accepted. Members feel free to share thoughts and ideas.

Performing: Members are productive and work for the common goal of the group. Interpersonal relations drive activities and results (Tuckman, 1965).

Adjourning: The team dissolves because the tasks have been completed and the goals achieved (Tuckman & Jensen, 1977).

During **forming**, the team members discover themselves and want to preserve their uniqueness or individuality. The goals and tasks for the team are offered, and individuals establish why they may have been selected for the team and how they can contribute. The focus is on individual interests, and testing comes in the form of establishing acceptable behaviors. The exchange of information is high as the team members establish ground rules and size each other up. As the team forms, selection of content experts and recognition of those who have implemented solutions in the past is common practice. Attention to different problem-solving styles and ensuring equal numbers of sensing/thinking versus intuitive/feeling members is key. This will benefit the group in the performing stage (but may be a source of conflict expressed in the storming stage). The team leader or project manager develops the explicit norm of constructive conflict by addressing disagreement, multiple definitions, minority opinions, the role of the "devil's advocate," and a "group wins" psychology (Antai-Otong, 2013; Bennett & Gadlin, 2012; Danna, 2013; Walters, 2012).

In the **storming** stage, members of the group jockey for position, control, and influence. Competition becomes apparent, and leadership struggles ensue. The honeymoon phase of orientation has lifted, and work requirements become evident. Resistance to team influence emerges, and intrateam conflict may arise. During this stage, team members have low levels of trust and often display anger and resentment. While turf battles may ensue, the foundations for trust and respect may be further developed during this stage as a result of how conflicts are resolved. The leader supports the team by assisting with assignments, team roles, and conflict resolution and abiding by the ground rules that were developed in the forming stage (Antai-Otong, 2013; Bennett & Gadlin, 2012, Danna, 2013; Walters, 2012).

During **norming**, team cohesion develops as roles and norms are established to promote decision-making through consensus. Members have a common understanding of the opportunity to reach team goals, and there is openness to alternative definitions and multiple views. Morale and trust are high, and negativity is suppressed.

Open communication during this stage facilitates constructive discussions and the sharing of personal and professional insights (Antai-Otong, 2013; Danna, 2013; Walters, 2012).

In the **performing stage** phase, team members work with deep involvement, greater disclosure, and unity. Bound together by common goals, productivity is high, and team synergy is evident as members rely on the talents of the team members to accomplish work. Loyalty to the team is evident, and efforts revolve around quality of team product. This is the phase where work is completed, and the leader may be less involved (Antai-Otong, 2013; Danna, 2013; Walters, 2012).

In the **adjourning stage**, team tasks and goals have been completed. The outcomes of the work often lead to self-evaluation by the team, both on an individual and collective basis. Some team members may experience sadness and mourning related to the absence of team interaction, routine, and sense of purpose (Antai-Otong, 2013; Danna, 2013; Walters, 2012).

The stages of team development are described as if sequential in nature. However, due to various factors, team development is not always linear. Phases may be repeated, interrupted, or skipped. With the entering of a new team member, the departure of a team member, new leadership, or revised goals and deliverables, the team may shift to an earlier or later stage to find new equilibrium along a continuum of performance (Antai-Otong, 2013; Danna, 2013; Walters, 2012).

As a project or program manager, having an understanding and awareness of these stages helps explain team member behaviors across the lifespan of the team. This knowledge prompts proactive approaches in guiding interprofessional teams composed of individuals with diverse backgrounds (educationally) and experiences (in terms of tenure and previous work on teams) to work through each developmental milestone appropriately. For example, recognizing that conflict during certain phases can actually bring harmony and productivity, the project manager who understands storming as a developmental stage can channel team conflict into positive energy and high performance. If the conflicts arise and persist in the performing stage, the project manager might intervene using a different approach that relies on the established interpersonal relationships of the team members to find a resolution (Walters, 2012; Antai-Otong, 2013; Tuckman, 1965). Overall, when seeking to create synergistic interprofessional teams that are dedicated to effective project planning, management, and person-centered programs, the project manager remains focused on ensuring that the team reaches the performing stage where team members are most productive.

▶ Building an Effective Team

Building a team is critical to the success of any project and often is the first challenge of executives, sponsors, and team leaders. Critical success of the compiled team members resides in the selection process, as each individual team member can provide knowledge, insight, and energy to the accomplishment of work or become an obstacle in attaining project goals.

Central to team selection are diversity, the attitude and skill of contributors, the ability of the team leader to build trust, and the balance between differing viewpoints and conflict management (Bennett & Gadlin, 2012). A shared purpose, mutual goals, and professional knowledge and maturity embodied in emotionally intelligent participants are desired. However, contrarians and novices are also needed. Likewise, those who know the process should work alongside those who indirectly contribute to the process and those impacted by the outcomes of the process. Selection criteria often starts with the role or position someone holds in an organization or the skillset the participant would contribute. Coupling this with a team inventory of desired attributes related to communication, flexibility, openness to differing ideas, and motivation can enhance the selection process to support achievement of desired outcomes (Bennett & Gadlin, 2012; Ryan, 2017).

Danna (2013) identified six rules to synergy and team building that are pivotal to interprofessional team effectiveness. The six rules are as follows:

1. Define a clear purpose. All team members must clearly be knowledgeable about the reason they are coming together. They must also be able to articulate the goals, objectives, and purpose of the team.

2. Actively listen. Each team member must be focused on each individual and listen to what is being said. Active listening is not judgmental and means being completely absorbed and attentive to the speaker.

3. Maintain honesty. Each team member must be objective in providing feedback to the speaker. No one should make the speaker feel belittled or that his or her view is not correct or important.

4. Demonstrate compassion. Each team member should listen in a caring manner to the other's viewpoint.

5. Commit to resolution of conflicts. Each team member must agree to disagree even though his or her view or opinions are not the same. Team members must work toward a common understanding and acceptance of the issue at hand.

6. Be flexible. Each team member must be open and flexible to another individual's perspective. Everyone works together to accomplish the goal or objective.

▶ Barriers to Team Effectiveness

While each of us enters a team with hope and anticipation, there are times when barriers arise that decrease the effectiveness of teams. Common pitfalls include an inability to trust or rely on team members, fear, unresolved conflict, lack of commitment, low standards, and the avoidance of accountability, as well as attention to personal gain rather than the results of the team. Each of these pitfalls can be avoided with effective leadership (Ulrich & Crider, 2017). To begin, the project or program manager's role is to assist the team in developing trusting relationships by demonstrating reliance on the team members to overcome limitations of knowledge, skills, or abilities that may be demonstrated by an individual team member. The team leader can demonstrate vulnerability and call on the members of the team to step forward to fill gaps. Fear and fear of conflict require team leaders to support constructive debates and demonstrate the ability to manage it by establishing group norms for dealing with issues in a manner that is respectful to all team members (Bennett & Gadlin, 2012; Ulrich & Crider, 2017).

When team members avoid taking a clear position on issues, the project or program manager must work with the team to provide critical information and a mechanism that considers all points of view before team decisions are made. Similarly, a lack of accountability can be countered by assisting the team to focus on goals, continually tracking team progress, and communicating frequently with the team through meetings and status reports.

Finally, inattention to the results of the team can be minimized through the selection of measures that clearly define success for the team effort (not individual interests) and the development of a tracking mechanism to monitor team progress. Success and failures must be equally shared within the team and used to reinforce progress toward goal achievement (Agency for Healthcare Research and Quality [AHRQ], 2015; Ulrich & Crider, 2017).

▶ Communication Processes Supporting Teamwork

The use of standardized communication tools to support teamwork amid complex healthcare systems has been explored in the literature as a means to improve decision-making and increase safety (AHRQ, 2015; Stewart & Hand, 2017). Strategies include the use of techniques such as **brainstorming**, nominal grouping, and **SBAR communication**.

Brainstorming sessions are used to generate a large number of ideas through interaction among team members. In this strategy, the objective of the brainstorming is established and is often directly related to the team goals. One individual is selected to record ideas (generally on a board or flip chart) to avoid duplications. Individuals in the group then call out ideas until all ideas are exhausted and, conversely, no new ideas emerge. The essential rules of brainstorming are that everyone participates and that no discussion, critique, or evaluation of the ideas takes place during the session. Following the creative thinking session, each idea is clarified to facilitate subsequent discussion on feasibility (Goldenberg & Wiley, 2011; Levine, Alexander, Wright, & Higgins, 2015).

In a similar manner, the nominal group process begins with the establishment of an objective but proceeds with each member generating his or her own list of possible solutions. When sufficient time has been allowed, members take turns calling out their ideas to the group. As with the brainstorming session, ideas are not discussed until all have been presented, and clarification occurs only after the team's entire list of ideas has been compiled (McMillan et al., 2014).

Once ideas are generated using brainstorming or nominal group processes, the team can then proceed to reduce the number of ideas on the list by voting to eliminate ideas that are not feasible, identifying items that may be readily implemented (low-hanging fruit), and ranking/ordering related alternatives. Once individual team members rank each idea, then idea percentage distributions or average score calculations can be performed to determine the degree of agreement among team members. Clarification and discussion of the internal strengths and weaknesses within the organization as well as external opportunities and threats outside the organization that currently or potentially support or mitigate actualization of the idea can be undertaken by the team and is referred to as a SWOT analysis. Additionally, an affinity diagram, in which ideas are written on cards and placed randomly on a table or chart, can be generated. Like or related ideas are then organized by the silently working team members. When cards are no longer being moved, the team then discusses the ideas and generates a title for each grouping. Each method is useful in exploring alternative plans of action toward goal attainment.

An additional strategy, SBAR communication, was developed at Kaiser Permanente and is among the techniques useful in teamwork for communicating essential information using a standardized format (Stewart & Hand, 2017). In this strategy, communication is provided using the format of situation, background, assessment, and recommendation (SBAR). The communication begins with a brief summary outline describing the situation. This is followed by background information about the situation or the context of the issue. The assessment component presents a statement of what the individual has identified as the problem and is followed by a recommendation of what corrective action is needed. Originally developed to facilitate communication between nurses and physicians, the use of a standardized format within team communication dynamics provides a succinct method of communicating information rapidly.

The work of a team to improve processes can be both challenging and rewarding. Effective leadership is facilitated through the use of structures and tools to ensure participation by all members of the team.

▶ Teamwork Strategies

Deliberate and distinct strategies to improve communication, define accountability, and establish routines have gained attention, in large part driven from the analysis of errors and their root causes and a commitment to improving quality, safety, effectiveness, and efficiency recommendations from the IOM (1999, 2001).

▶ TeamSTEPPs

Created by the Agency for Healthcare Research and Quality and the Department of Defense, this evidence-based teamwork model was developed to describe necessary skills and behaviors for team outcomes. The model includes skills for leadership, mutual support, situation monitoring, and communication. Attention to team composition, leadership, communication strategies and skills, standardization, and shared purpose underpin effectiveness. Feedback cycles are used with specific tools for communication to plan, deliver care, and evaluate care. Tools such as briefings, team huddles, and SBAR communication are the foundation from which fewer errors and improved outcomes flow (AHRQ, n.d.-a, n.d.-b, 2015; Danna, 2013).

▶ Synergy and Creativity

While the essence of project or program management is a systematic and disciplined approach to leading people through change and the completion of tasks, it also provides the opportunity to bring new ideas, relationships, and enthusiasm to an organization. The confidence of the team leader in navigating pitfalls and deliberately bringing people through the achievement of milestones is expected. What may be overlooked is the opportunity for creativity and transformation, often displayed by teams led by seasoned project managers. In times of great change or uncertainty, it is easy to draw from past experiences and conform to rules or practices that brought success in the past. **Appreciative inquiry**, coupled with project management skills and quality improvement structures, can move teams from transactional interactions to transformational results and warrants attention given the expectations placed upon us during the era of health reform.

While difficult to define, synergy is a product of effective teams, and the experience is commonly cited by team members as one of the benefits and personal satisfiers of working in a highly effective team. As individuals become members of a team and successfully work through the developmental stages, an energy, respect, and anticipation of positive outcomes buoys the members as they experience the benefits of productively working well together. While sharing experiences and implementing change, team members' synergistic influence is expanded by inciting enthusiasm and the spirit of possibility with individuals outside the work team (Gottlieb & Gottlieb, 2017; Lewis, Fitzgerald, & Zulkiewicz, 2017).

In consideration of professional development and team identity, synergy is experienced by those working in teams and is often described as growth derived from relationships, feedback, and insights gained from the experience. Attributes that contribute to synergy come through the interactions of team members supported by active listening, contributing, motivation, and cognition (Porter-O'Grady & Malloch, 2015). A team-level phenomenon of synergy has been described as an unconscious process of the team that manifests in individual team member actions that create collective positive or negative outcomes very different from the outcomes that would have been achieved by simply adding up the contributions of the individuals. Part of the synergy comes from the active listening and openness of team members as they explore options that may have been dismissed by an individual, lending to the creativity. Another part of the synergy comes from the self-correcting function of teams to counteract undesired outcomes and position the team to use individual and team creative assets.

▶ Appreciative Inquiry

While often thought of as a strategic lever for leadership and change, appreciative inquiry (AI) has applications relevant to project and program management in light of the need to preserve clinical outcomes and quality metrics. At its core, AI is the art and practice of asking questions that strengthen a systems capacity to apprehend, anticipate, and heighten positive potential. Focused on what *is* working rather than what is not, it shifts thinking away from our typical "what is not working" focus and guides us to greater acknowledgment and preservation of those things that do work well. Rather than finding deficits and gaps, AI brings attention to strengths within teams or organizations and those things that can be replicated.

Cooperrider's (1990) seminal work in AI describes four stages: discovery, dream, design, and destiny. **Discovery** is the mobilization of the team or system into a positive change core. The **dream** stage occurs when a transparent, results-oriented vision is created through discovering potential and questions that provide a higher purpose. **Design** occurs when possibilities are realized with regard to the ideal state and people feel capable of expanding the positive core, making new dreams and concepts. **Destiny** evolves from the strengthening of the positive capabilities and capacities of the system, building hope and momentum focused on deeper purpose. Because members of the organization feel safe and energized, a space for learning, adjustment, and improvisation is created (Thomas & Roussel, 2013).

AI is an intervention that heightens imagination and **innovation** by mobilizing a spirit of inquiry. The language of AI is different from our current state, given that critical analysis and identification of what is not working often take more time and attention than the celebrations of what is working.

Hubbard (1998) views AI as a conscious evolution for realities in the new century. It recognizes social construction focusing on metaphor, ways of knowing, and language producing a generative theory and advancement in action research. AI has been used in organizational development practice, as part of strategic planning, and as a framework to move from problem-based management to transformative leadership and human development (Thomas & Roussel, 2013).

▶ Transformational Leadership

Given the need for engagement, honesty, innovation, trust, creativity, and recognition of things valued by members of teams, AI as a framework to generate solutions merits consideration. Underlying the success of AI are strong leaders with clarity, vision, and the ability to influence the thinking of others. **Transformational leadership** has been recognized as a style of leadership that extends beyond transactions. Transformational leadership includes a change or transformation of both the leader and the follower when leaders broaden, extend, and elevate the interests of employees, generate awareness and acceptance of the purposes and mission of the team, and stir employees to look beyond their own self-interests for the good of the group (Bennis & Nanus, 1985; Roussel & Ratcliffe, 2013). In this way, leaders are agents of change who influence and inspire others and then are also changed.

Transformational leaders motivate followers to perform beyond normal expectations by transforming their thoughts and attitudes and by enlisting the vital support of the vision while striving for its fulfillment. This is accomplished through attributed charisma or modeling behaviors that gain admiration and trust; inspirational motivation or the ability to envision and articulate a future; intellectual stimulation involving questioning assumptions and reframing problems from a new perspective; and individualized consideration by delegation and empowerment while attending to individual needs, abilities, and aspirations (Avolio & Bass, 2002; Bass, 1990). The theory of transformational leadership implies people need a sense of mission that extends beyond transactions and interpersonal relationships. This is especially true in health care, where the speed of and demand for change often exceed our perceived capacity.

For project and program managers, transformational leadership offers a framework that promotes the synergistic interprofessional teamwork required for effective project planning, management, and person-centered care. Empowerment of others, clarity in vision, and expectations of transformative change through the leadership of teams generate synergy around creative possibilities not previously considered. Transformative leadership brings extraordinary results through its capacity to influence others, build trust, and support teams as they press through their work to accomplish goals. Aspiring to become a transformational leader is within the reach of project and program managers.

▶ Innovation

Much has been published on the need to hardwire evidence-based practices. Recently, attention has shifted from evidence to innovation. Porter-O'Grady and Malloch (2015) pointedly stated, "Innovation is not merely a process. It is a dynamic. Innovation gives new meaning and direction and challenges the historic, the expected, and the routine.

It calls for innovators to adopt an attitude that reflects that all work processes and activities are subject to the discipline of constant inquiry and reassessment" (p. 155).

The challenge for the interprofessional team is not how to generate new ideas and opportunities but to make innovation a deeply entrenched aptitude and competency in any project endeavor (Gibson, 2014). The innovative project team should ensure that the integrity and sustainability of the projects' outcomes are adaptable to the changing supply and demands of both the internal and external environment and that the collective interest of the organization is advanced through those outcomes. Producing value in a singular innovative project can create opportunities for additional value-based opportunistic projects. Sustained project outcomes and effective teams are the goal of and standard for high-functioning innovative systems where a culture of innovation is valued and respected. Missed opportunities occur daily in clinical settings and life in general. Harnessing the energy and talents of an interprofessional team will turn missed opportunities into an innovative pipeline that produces high-quality, safe, and effective outcomes that benefit varying populations and communities.

▶ Summary

- Effective project and program management is dependent on the ability to facilitate teams and guide them to successful goal attainment.
- Time spent in understanding team dynamics is well spent, followed by leadership development to support and sustain trust, satisfaction, and accomplishment of goals by creating a space where curiosity and innovation are the norm.
- The five stages of team development, forming, storming, norming, performing, and adjourning, are the platform on which effective teams can be built to perform.
- The challenge to synergistic, interprofessional teams is to adopt an aptitude of innovation that is disciplined, constantly inquiring, and reassessing.
- Strategies directed toward building trust, effective communication, curiosity, and innovation will serve organizations moving through the demands placed on the industry in care delivery redesign.

Reflection Questions

1. You are assigned to lead a project to reduce readmissions to your hospital. The CEO has identified that the first priority is to prevent unnecessary readmissions from skilled nursing facilities and home care agencies that your health system owns. Whom would you request to be on this team, and why? What would be your first steps?

2. You have been asked to step in and chair a subcommittee of the Quality and Safety Committee of the Board. The subcommittee you will chair has been charged to create a patient safety program, and the leader of this group has been on leave for 3 months. The trends by unit show increasing injury fall rates and increases in medication errors despite bar-code scanning. After reviewing the team charter and the outcomes dashboard for the work of this subcommittee, you realize that the team has stalled and that the metrics/measures of success have not changed for more than a year despite meeting monthly. You know you'll need to make some changes to achieve the team charge. You've been asked to write your plan for a meeting with the CEO and CNO tomorrow.

What would you include in your plan? What recommendations might you make regarding selection of new team members or disbanding this team and starting with new members? To manage expectations, what would you emphasize to the senior executives in terms of the team composition, timing, and future meetings?

3. You have been asked to join a newly created organizational team tasked to create the strategy and processes to increase department-specific innovations to fulfill the Triple Aim. As you listened to the discussion, you walked away feeling like the team didn't have a clear definition of what innovation is. You decide to call the team chair to meet for lunch so that you can learn about how "innovation" will be defined. Knowing what you do about the discipline and rigor involved in project and team leadership, who else in the organization would you want to talk to before the next meeting? What approach might you take with the team to generate ideas? What resources would you tap to assess the organization's past successes with change and innovation?

References

Agency for Healthcare Research and Quality (AHRQ). (n.d.-a). *TeamSTEPPS national implementation*. Retrieved from http://teamstepps.ahrq.gov/about-2cl_3.htm

Agency for Healthcare Research and Quality (AHRQ). (n.d.-b). *TeamSTEPPS: Strategies and tools to enhance performance and patient safety*. Retrieved from http://www.ahrq.gov/professionals /education/curriculum-tools/teamstepps/index.html

Agency for Healthcare Research and Quality (AHRQ). (2015). *TeamSTEPPS 2.0*. Retrieved from https://www.ahrq.gov/teamstepps/instructor/fundamentals/index.html

Antai-Otong, D. (2013). Effective communication and team collaboration. In J. L. Harris, L. Roussel, & P. Thomas (Eds.), *Initiating and sustaining the clinical nurse leader role: A practical guide* (2nd ed.). Burlington, MA: Jones & Bartlett Learning.

Armstead, C., Bierman, D., Bradshaw, P., Martin, T., & Wright, K. (2016). Groups vs. teams: Which one are you leading? *Nurse Leader, 14*(3), 179–182. http://dx.doi.org/10.1016/j.mnl.2016.03.006

Avolio, B., & Bass, B. (2002). *Developing potential across a full range of leadership: Cases on transactional and transformational leadership*. Mahwah, NJ: Lawrence Erlbaum Associates, Publishers.

Bass, B. (1990). *Bass & Stogdill's handbook of leadership: Theory, research, and managerial applications* (3rd ed). New York: NY: The Free Press.

Bennett, L., & Gadlin, H. (2012). Collaboration and team science. *Journal of Investigative Medicine, 60*(5), 768. http://dx.doi.org/10.2310/JIM.0b013e318250871d

Bennis, W., & Nanus, B. (1985). *Leadership: The strategies for taking charge*. New York, NY: Harper & Row.

Braithewaite, J. (2015). Bridging gaps to promote networked care between teams and groups in health delivery systems: A systematic review of non-health literature. *BMJ Open; London, 5*(9), 1–12.

Cooperrider, D. (1990). Positive image, positive action: The affirmative basis of organization. In S. Srivastva & D. L. Cooperrider (Eds.), *Appreciative management and leadership* (pp. 91–125). San Francisco, CA: Jossey-Bass.

Danna, D. (2013). Organizational structure and analysis. In L. Roussel (Ed.), *Management and leadership for nurse administrators* (6th ed., pp. 213–307). Burlington, MA: Jones & Bartlett Learning.

Gibson, R. (2014). *The no. 1 challenge to innovation*. Retrieved from http://www.innovationexcellence .com/blog,2014/09/14/the-no-1-challenge-to-innovation.

Goldenberg, O., & Wiley, J. (2011). Quality, conformity, and conflict: Questioning the assumptions of Osborn's brainstorming technique. *Journal of Problem Solving, 3*(2), 96–118.

Gottlieb, L., & Gottlieb, B. (2017). Strengths-based nursing: A process for implementing a philosophy into practice. *Journal of Family Nursing, 23*(3), 319–340.

Hewitt, G., Sims, S., & Harris, R. (2014). Using realist synthesis to understand the mechanisms of interprofessional teamwork in health and social care. *Journal of Interprofessional Care, 28*(6), 501–506.

Hubbard, B. (1998). *Conscious evolution: Awakening the power of our social potential*. Novato, CA: New World Library.

Institute of Medicine. (1999). *To err is human: Building a safer health system*. Washington, DC: National Academies Press.

Institute of Medicine Committee on Quality of Health Care in America. (2001). *Crossing the quality chasm: A new health system for the 21st century*. Washington, DC: National Academy Press.

Interprofessional Education Collaborative Expert Panel. (2011). *Core competencies for interprofessional collaborative practice: Report of an expert panel*. Washington, D.C.: Interprofessional Education Collaborative.

Levine, J., Alexander, K., Wright, A., & Higgins, E. (2015). Group brainstorming: When regulatory nonfit enhances performance. *Group Processes & Intergroup Relations, 19*(2), 257–271.

Lewis, M., Fitzgerald, T., & Zulkiewicz, B. (2017). Identifying synergies in multilevel interventions: The convergence strategy. *Health Education & Behavior, 44*(2), 236–244.

McMillan, S., Kelly, F., Sav, A., Kendall, E., King, M., Whitty, J., & Wheeler, A. (2014). Using the nominal group technique: How to analyse across multiple groups. *Health Services & Outcomes Research Methodology, 14*(3), 92–108.

Mueller, S. (2016). Transdisciplinary coordination and delivery of care. *Seminars in Oncology Nursing, 32*(2), 154–163.

Nancarrow, S., Booth, A., Ariss, S., Smith, T., Enderby, P., & Roots, A. (2013). Ten principles of good interdisciplinary team work. *Human Resources for Health, 11*(19). http://dx.doi .org/10.1186/1478-4491-11-19

O'Toole, M. (2003). *Miller-Keane encyclopedia and dictionary of medicine, nursing, and allied health*, (7th ed.). Amsterdam, Netherlands: Elsevier.

Porter-O'Grady, T., & Malloch, K. (2015). *Quantum leadership: Building better partnerships for sustainable health* (4th ed.). Burlington, MA: Jones & Bartlett Learning.

Project Management Institute. (2013). *A guide to project management body of knowledge (PMBOK guide)* (5th ed.). Newtown Square, PA: Author.

Robert Wood Johnson Foundation & Institute of Medicine. (2010). *The future of nursing: Leading change, advancing health*. Retrieved from https://www.nap.edu/resource/12956/Future-of -Nursing-2010-Report-Brief.pdf

Roussel, L., & Ratcliffe, C. (2013). Transformational leadership and evidence-based management in a changing world. In L. Roussel (Ed.), *Management and leadership for nurse administrators* (6th ed., pp. 729–756). Burlington, MA: Jones & Bartlett Learning.

Ryan, S. (2017). Promoting effective teamwork in the healthcare setting. *Nursing Standard, 31*(30), 52. http://dx.doi.org/10.7748/ns.2017.e10726

Stewart, K., & Hand, K. (2017). SBAR, communication, and patient safety: An integrated literature review. *Medsurg Nursing, 26*(5), 297–305.

Thomas, P., & Roussel, L. (2013). Clinical nurse leadership: Creating the vision. In J. L. Harris, L. Roussel, & P. Thomas (Eds.) *Initiating and sustaining the clinical nurse leader role: A practical guide* (2nd ed., pp. 481–510). Burlington, MA: Jones & Bartlett Learning.

Tuckman, B. (1965). Developmental sequence in small groups. *Psychological Bulletin, 63*, 384–399.

Tuckman, B., & Jensen, M. (1977). Stages of small group development revisited. *Groups and Organizational Studies, 2*, 419–427.

Ulrich, B., & Crider, N. M. (2017). Using teams to improve outcomes and performance. *Nephrology Nursing Journal, 44*(2), 141–151.

Walters, S. (2012). Team power and synergy: Project planning and program management essentials. In J. L. Harris, L. Roussel, S. Walters, & C. Dearman (Eds.), *Project planning and management: A guide for CNLs, DNPs and nurse executives* (pp. 39–50). Burlington, MA: Jones & Bartlett Learning.

Zaccagnini, M. & White, K. (2014). *The doctor of nursing practice essentials; a new model for advanced practice nursing*, 2nd ed, Burlington MA: Jones & Bartlett.

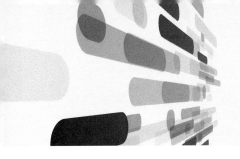

Case Exemplar

▶ Case Study 1

Emotional Intelligence: A Catalyst for Interprofessional Team Success

Margaret Mitchell

All behavior has purpose and consequences, whether recognized at a given moment or at a later time during self-reflection. Failure to recognize how one reacts to situations and subsequent interactions with others can be a detriment to individual and team success. Interactions among team members drive outcomes and successful change. If a member of a team is resistant and/or reactive during a situation and is unaware of this behavior, the entire team may suffer. A project's potential outcomes may therefore be unattainable or significantly reduced. The interactions, relationships, and emotional intelligence of team members become vital to individual (evolutionary) or team (revolutionary) change in today's chaotic healthcare environment. If these are overlooked, opportunities for both team synergy and the notion of mindfulness are reduced, if not lost. Being mindful of recurring situations, past reactions, and emotions can only improve the odds for interprofessional team synergy and success.

Numerous authors have recognized the importance of one's emotional intelligence as a determinant for achieving personal and team excellence (Bradberry & Graves, 2009; George, 2000; Goleman, 1998). According to Goleman, emotional intelligence determines the potential for learning the practical skills of emotional competence. Appreciation and governance of one's emotions and those of the team can help alleviate team conflict as team activities and interprofessional projects evolve (George, 2000). Bradberry and Graves (2009) and Goleman (1998) advocate for the reinvestment in beliefs and values as an opportunity to redirect disruptive impulses that are prone to suspend judgment and to think before acting. Failing to handle or even consider one's actions or consider the feelings of others limits team synergy and any sustainable outcomes. This may further diminish the commitment and motivation of any team in the immediate and long-range future (Porter-O'Grady & Malloch, 2015).

Throughout one's career, nurses and other professionals are required to interact with one another. Observing how individuals respond to members of their individual discipline, especially nurses, can be especially enlightening, as the phrase "we eat our own" is commonplace when listening to nurses in conversation. Being mindful of how another nurse responds to a new graduate nurse can be directly attributed to one's emotional intelligence and can directly impact this relationship. A negative response or action can create conflict, and when individuals are unaware of their own negativity or reactivity in such a situation, this behavior may be observed in interactions with others.

While there are no guarantees to changing how one reacts to any situation or crisis, thought leaders have offered several insights into enhancing one's emotional intelligence and potentials for effective and sustainable interprofessional team synergy (Goleman, 1998; Porter-O'Grady & Malloch, 2015). These include the following:

- Openness to novel ideas
- Valuing the knowledge and expertise of others
- Compassion
- Resilience
- Passion toward accomplishing a team goal
- Impulse control

The value of emotional intelligence advances a team's function and outcomes. Team members who are attuned to self and use their emotional intelligence can be beneficial to outcomes and sustained success. Being open to serendipitous and developing influences that occur unexpectedly is a hallmark of an emotionally intelligent team member and an effective team. Such influences can improve care delivery and advance health care in the 21st century and beyond.

Reflection Questions

1. Which of your personal strengths and attributes advance team functioning?
2. How are these attributes used in your daily practice environment?
3. What skills or abilities do you want to develop to become a more effective interdisciplinary or interprofessional team member? Why did you select these skills or abilities?

References

Bradberry, T., & Graves, J. (2009). *Emotional intelligence 2.0*. San Diego, CA: TalentSmart.

George, J. (2000). Emotions and leadership: The role of emotional intelligence. *Human Relations, 53*(8), 1027–1055.

Goleman, D. (1998). *Working with emotional intelligence*. New York, NY: Bantam.

Porter-O'Grady, T., & Malloch, K. (2015). *Quantum leadership: Building better partnerships for sustainable health* (4th ed.). Burlington, MA: Jones & Bartlett Learning.

CHAPTER 8

Managing the Interprofessional Project Team

James L. Harris
Kathryn M. Ward-Presson

CHAPTER OBJECTIVES

1. Recognize the key elements of managing interprofessional teams during projects in a competitive and chaotic healthcare environment.
2. Explore the importance of a common language shared by clinical and administrative project planners and managers.
3. Translate the characteristics of coaching interprofessional teams in the planning, initiating, and evaluating phases of projects.
4. Describe the needs of interprofessional teams and the significance of team leadership in maintaining continuous performance given the mandates imposed by accrediting agencies and stakeholders.
5. Identify key areas associated with measuring team leader effectiveness.

KEY TERMS

Collaboration
Communication
Interdisciplinary team
Interprofessional team
Language

Organizational culture
Performance
Professionalism
Team leader effectiveness
Team synergy

ROLES

Coach   Leader

PROFESSIONAL VALUES

Quality

CORE COMPETENCIES

Assessment   Evaluating
Communication   Innovation
Coordination   Interpersonal relationships
Design   Leadership
Diversity   Management
Emotional intelligence   Policy management

▶ Introduction

Health care remains at a crossroads, as patients' medical conditions become increasingly more complex, reimbursement and regulatory mandates expand and intensify, and knowledge emerges from a series of catalyzing changes that challenge care delivery globally. As innovative quality projects are planned and applied, engagement of **interprofessional team** members and their continuous management are vital to success. Speaking a common **language** and understanding the meaning of each term and concept translates into significant outcomes and **team synergy**. Knowledge gleaned from projects requires mobilization of the evidence through continuous **communication** and consciousness-raising if innovation is to be sustained (Crisp, 2014). Healthcare organizations have unprecedented opportunities to assume the challenges to innovate and leverage knowledge on many levels. When various disciplines engage in interprofessional projects, education, and collaborative practice, high-quality, safe, and efficient care is realized as evidence-based knowledge is spread (Interprofessional Education Collaborative [IPEC] Expert Panel, 2011; World Health Organization [WHO], 2013).

This chapter discusses the essentials in managing interprofessional teams that are engaged in clinical and quality projects and emphasizes the importance of using a common language in all phases of projects, their management, and collaborative efforts. The value of coaching interprofessional project teams is also addressed as a means to capitalize on team **performance** given the changing healthcare landscape being driven by new and existing accrediting, regulatory, and stakeholder demands.

▶ Interprofessional Teams: Overview and Management

Achieving optimal outcomes is a hallmark of any team effort. However, sustaining those outcomes requires **professionalism**, ongoing engagement, commitment, collaborative interprofessional practice, and management. Each professional must work independently and in parallel to one another. Drinka and Clark (2000) reiterated the need to function interdependently as solutions are generated collaboratively. The concepts of interprofessional teams and collaborative practice are not foreign ideas to healthcare professionals. Zaccagnini and White (2014), for example, support the notion that effective interprofessional teamwork and **collaboration** include not just vested professionals but other stakeholders and team members from various disciplines. A well-orchestrated and assembled project team may require the inclusion of patients as well as professionals from technology, health policy management, and library science. Rigorously aligning and integrating the needs and interests of individuals collectively creates a transformative connection. Ideas can be generated, shared, and communicated toward a defined aim. This approach can guide projects, add value, and create avenues for managing processes and conflicts that may arise during any project team effort. Value, whether directly or indirectly, indicates growth or improvement occurring within the team, system, or project (Dunevitz, 1997).

To provide a context for the remainder of this chapter and throughout the text, it is important to distinguish between interprofessional teams and **interdisciplinary teams** given that both terms are used—sometimes interchangeably—in the literature. These terms actually have quite different meanings. Zaccagnini and White (2014) distinguish "interprofessional" as signaling the inclusion of representatives from a particular discipline or knowledge branch with differing experiences, education, values, roles, and expectations. By comparison, "interdisciplinary" is more specific to a particular discipline. Generally, "interprofessional" is associated with a broader definition and context as related to projects, collaborative efforts, and their management.

The rapidity of change in the healthcare industry has necessitated support of understanding and integrating management and leadership, as interprofessional project teams have proved able to generate novel approaches for meeting the increasing demands made by consumers and the healthcare industry itself. Managing a successful team that is dedicated to improvement and practice change requires the development of reciprocal trust and continuous interpersonal relationships among team members (Kouzes & Pozner, 2007). If time is not allowed for teams to progress through developmental stages, managing the team will be almost impossible, and the potential gains from a team's synergy will be lost. In 1965, Tuckman proposed a model for group stages that has proved valuable in understanding a team's development. A final stage was later identified that further supported team synergy (Tuckman, 2001). These five stages—forming, storming, norming, performing, and adjourning—are discussed next.

Forming is the initial stage in which the team comes together for the purpose of completing a defined project aim. During this stage, trust is essential as the team members get to know one another, form interpersonal relationships, clearly articulate the group's aim, and further define their roles and responsibilities.

In the *storming* stage, team trust has not fully developed, and conflicts may arise due to differing disciplines, opinions, and lived experiences. Communication and directly approaching conflicts are essential actions by the team leader at this stage. The complexity of individual differences, gender, culture, ethnicity, language, and emotions can limit communication, however, such that further conflicts may ensue. Conflicts are frequent when there is resistance to change. Some individuals may be satisfied with the status quo and threatened by change; they require the leader to openly address this stance lest opportunities to meet a goal or aim and learn from others are diminished. Unresolved conflict reduces productivity, lowers team morale, and is costly (Chinn, 2008; Feldman, 2008; Patterson, Grenny, McMillian, & Switzler, 2002).

The emotional intelligence of team members and the team leader is of utmost importance during the storming stage. Emotions can become a barrier to moving forward as a productive team to accomplish the specific aim (McCallin & Bamford, 2007). Emotional intelligence (EI) is a valuable leadership attribute in terms of the awareness of the role played by emotion in communication, rapport building, and motivation. According to Goleman (1998), EI determines the potential for learning the practical skills of emotional competence and is divided into five realms:

- Self-awareness: The ability to recognize and understand one's emotions, moods, and drives, as well as the effects on others.
- Self-regulation: The ability to handle emotions so that they do not interfere with project work yet to be completed.
- Motivation: The desire to engage in work beyond personal reasons.
- Empathy: The ability to understand the emotions of others.
- Social skill: Skill in relationship management and network building needed to meet a common understanding and rapport. (Goleman 1998)

As an attribute of the leader, EI is credited with contributing to many successes and often plays a more significant role than cognitive abilities as the project team progresses in its work (Goleman, Boyzatsis, & McKee, 2002).

Norming is the next stage, where team identity begins to develop. During this stage, open dialogue is promoted in which ideas and differing insights are shared and accepted. The team leader needs to be alert to preventing groupthink at this point, as it could inhibit progression to the next stage.

As the *performing* stage matures, team loyalty and assets of team members are used to full benefit. Territorial differences by professionals need to be removed, as flexibility is a common indicator of the ability to accomplish the project's stated aim. Finally, in the *adjourning* stage, performance and progress are evaluated in terms of the outcomes.

Throughout each of these stages, a shared purpose, trust, respect and recognition, collaboration, shared responsibility, and mutual decision-making are markers for successful progression. Healthcare systems are complex, adaptive systems requiring flexibility, collaboration, use of a common language by team members, and responsibility for the ultimate project aim to be met and patient-centered care accomplished (Begun, Zimmerman, & Dooley, 2003).

▶ A Common Language: A Driver for Interprofessional Project Team Success

Interprofessional project teams are composed of individuals from varying backgrounds, both clinically and culturally. Developing and adopting a mutually agreed-upon common language and shared purpose can only benefit the project and functions as a driver for team success and measurable outcomes for future replication (Kouzes & Pozner, 2007).

Central to the team leader's role is understanding the communication preferences of various generations represented on the project team and the challenge to succeed. In a technology-driven environment, the challenge of making rapid changes and responding to identified issues may hinder a project team unless the communication preferences of various generations are considered and used to benefit the project aim (Martin & Tulgan, 2006). **TABLE 8-1** describes some of the communication preferences

TABLE 8-1 Communication Preferences by Generation		
Generation	**Spoken Preference**	**Written Preference**
Traditionalists (Birth years: 1900–1945)	Formal linear thinkers, direct and to the point, no foul or offensive language, no small talk, proper grammar.	Well organized, proper grammar and punctuation, to the point, like written communication for future reference.
Baby Boomers (Birth years: 1946–1964)	Like small talk to consensus and foster teamwork.	Written word for later reference and creation of paper trail preferred.
Generation X (Birth years: 1965–1980)	Informal and direct with little to no small talk. Focus is on what things mean for them.	Little preference for reading; desire concise bullet points with outcomes clearly delineated. Little focus on grammar and punctuation.
Millennials (Birth years: 1981–2000)	Prefer spoken communication if the message is very important; desire others to show respect through language spoken; prefer action verbs with important messages; desire use of language to portray visual pictures; not skilled at personal communication because of the technical ways of communicating used during their lifespan.	Use positive, respectful, motivational electronic communication style; portray pictures through language; use action verbs. May need direction or written communication formats.

by generation. Keeping these pointers in mind when leading and managing project teams will prove beneficial to a positive product.

Unintentional and various jargon used by project team members can also hinder the progress of the team. It is not uncommon to observe different disciplines or individuals with personal agendas from a specific discipline who have priorities that compete with the project aim. For example, on a pain management project team, different disciplines or individuals may differ in terms of their preferred pain assessment techniques, observations, and descriptors; in turn, these differences may create a barrier to accomplishing the aim of developing a mutually agreeable language and process for documenting and describing a patient's pain experience.

As noted previously, communication barriers are created when others do not comprehend the language, which then limits opportunities for mutual idea and knowledge sharing. Kaiser Permanente developed the standardized tool known as SBAR (situation, background, assessment, and recommendation) communication to deal with this risk. Interprofessional teams use the SBAR tool for discussion and solving patient problem situations; it provides a succinct method for ensuring team information exchange in a rapid cycle. Project teams also find this tool useful for achievement of project milestones (Leonard, Graham, & Bonacum, 2004).

Project teams may also benefit from other shared, common language as projects are envisioned and implemented. For example, the National Patient Safety Goals and the Institute of Medicine's (IOM) Six Safety Aims highlight contributions by interprofessional teams in achieving desired, measurable collaborative goals (IOM, 2001; The Joint Commission, 2018). Many projects today focus on quality, safety, efficiency, and opportunities in an effort to demonstrate sustainable outcomes with replicable measurement and generation of empirical data. Language included in Lean, Six Sigma, and other methodologies offers a sustainable means of engaging in projects that emphasize the continuum of care, care coordination, pay for performance, and at-risk contracting for payment (Naylor, 2012).

An organization's culture plays an important role in how information is communicated and language is used, and both of these factors influence every project plan and activity. **Organizational culture** also plays an important role in all healthcare processes and the interchanges between patients and providers. Organizations that engender ingenuity of project improvement teams and remove an entrenched "culture of blame" in favor of a "just culture" will prevail in these turbulent times. Notably, safer practices will follow when the just culture approach is adopted (Scott-Cawiezell, Jones, Moore, & Vojir, 2004). Just cultures foster supportive environments in which staff can questions practices, express concerns, and admit mistakes without punishment (Kennedy, 2016; Tucker, Nembhard, & Edmondson, 2007). A supportive environment is the cornerstone for a successful organization where employees are engaged and eager to be innovators (Hoying, 2017).

If an organization is able to promote interprofessional project teams that invest their efforts in advancing practice and creating empirical evidence, it is likely to have fewer incidents and system failures than an organization that holds on to the traditional "culture of blame" (Khatri, Brown, & Hicks, 2009). Incorporating the language of just culture and being true to its meaning will continuously foster positive team function and sustainability. Hence, high-reliability organizations are realized in which care is safe and errors are minimized while achieving exceptional performance in quality, safety, and efficacy (LaPorte, 2006).

▶ Coaching Interprofessional Project Teams

Teams are the driving force to success in any organization. Whether they form a functional team, a team of managers, or a specific project team, people collaboratively working together produce effective outcomes. As part of interprofessional team socialization, coaches assist members throughout all phases of a project. Coaches act as connectors who know lots of people. Their importance extends beyond the *number* of people they know to the *kinds* of people they know (Gladwell, 2002). A coach uses this information when working with teams to assist them in recognizing the value of all members and the importance of demonstrating interprofessional respect toward one another. Otherwise, the performance and productivity of a project suffer.

Hanson and Spross (2009) posit that a paradox of the current healthcare system is the existence of both incentives and disincentives for interprofessional team members and organizations to collaborate. Both the incentives and the disincentives play powerful roles, such that motivation to collaborate is eliminated by a counterforce. Recognizing this paradox will assist interprofessional project teams in seizing opportunities for strategic and sustainable collaboration in supportive environments.

Team coaching can be a powerful tool as teams work together to accomplish a specific aim. Coaching is a method used for support, encouragement, and career development (Finkelman & Kenner, 2010). Equally important is showing teams how to reduce conflict and improve working relationships for achievement of an identified aim.

Coaching a team requires this leader to focus on skills and interactions versus individual development. Interactions with team members and their communication are central to effective performance. One of the initial characteristics of a successful coach is understanding the team dynamics and translating this information throughout the phases of the project so as to attain the desired outcomes. Identifying how team members relate to one another is important for decision-making and productivity. Indeed, member behavioral assessments often prove beneficial for improving a team's productivity. As a coach, encouraging group discussion of behavioral assessments assists members to see one another differently, understand other people's perspectives, and adapt individual behavior for improved results. To realize this outcome, the team coach must ensure that a clear set of behavior expectations is mutually established and maintained to eliminate individual preferences that might otherwise obscure the project aim. Defining processes for team members to follow will support this endeavor.

Recognizing the need to evaluate reward and recognition systems and support individual development are the final roles of a team coach. When team members have personal goals that do not match with the goals of the team, problems may potentially arise. In such a case, the coach needs to identify sources of competing values and ensure that reward systems align correctly with individual performance. Being supportive of individual development is important for the coach as well, as members ideally will gain insights and attain new skills that ultimately benefit them individually in future team activities as well as the current project (Edmonson, 1999; Hall & Weaver, 2001).

In summary, Hackman and Wageman (2005, p. 283) suggest that team coaching will foster effectiveness only when four conditions are present:

1. The group performance processes that are key to performance effectiveness (i.e., effort, strategy, and knowledge and skill) are relatively unconstrained by task or organizational requirements.

2. The team is well designed, and the organizational context within which it operates supports rather than impedes teamwork.

3. Coaching behaviors focus on salient task performance processes rather than members' interpersonal relationships or on processes that are not under the team's control.

4. Coaching interventions are made at times when the team is ready for them and able to deal with them—that is, at the beginning for effort-related (motivational) interventions, near the midpoint for strategy-related (consultative) interventions, and at the end of a task cycle for (educational) interventions that address knowledge and skills. (Hackman and Wageman (2005, p. 283)

Reproduced with permission from The Academy of Management Review. Hackman, J. & Wageman, R. (2005). A Theory of Team Coaching. *The Academy of Management Review, 30*(2), 283; permission conveyed through Copyright Clearance Center, Inc.

▶ Leading Interprofessional Project Teams Based on Needs and Mandates

Despite widespread agreement in disciplines about the centrality of clinical experiences to knowledge acquisition, extensive findings about the teaching practices or learning opportunities that foster interprofessional healthcare teams' outcomes remain limited. Such knowledge will benefit acquisition of the knowledge and skills needed to design and implement interprofessional projects resulting in safe, quality care. The extent to which individuals are best positioned to lead effective clinical or administrative project teams reflects needs, competencies, and competing mandates.

The 21st-century technologies, accreditation standards, and stakeholder demands for teamwork, communication, and coordination rely heavily on evidence to inform processes and care delivery. Identifying the needs of interprofessional project teams highlights the importance of leading them to engage in continuous improvement. Likewise, leaders and teams who possess interprofessional competencies and understand the interrelationships between patients and the team will facilitate project completion and satisfaction of the mandates that often drive management actions and decisions (IPEC Expert Panel, 2011).

Leaders at all levels must be action oriented and are challenged to shape new clinical environments and create a culture that incorporates change. Unlike management that seeks to control and manage, leaders seek to create and inspire change (Kotter, 1990). This change will be influenced, managed, and ultimately evaluated as it spreads to other environments. The call to create environments and core competencies sensitive to interprofessional team needs, strengths, and cultural diversity recognizes this reality. Globalization has promoted team inclusivity and ethnic diversity, resulting in multiple improvements (American Association of Colleges of Nursing, 2015). But one may ask, why now, and which core competencies should be adopted and utilized that maximize leader performance and preference?

The Interprofessional Education Collaborative (IPEC) Practice Competencies panel is one group that has accepted the call to action and attempted to answer this question. This panel suggested the following steps as a response:

1. Create efforts across professions to ensure content is included in curricula.
2. Guide curricular development toward outcomes.

3. Provide foundations for a learning continuum across professions that embrace and engender lifelong learning.
4. Acknowledge that evaluation and empirical inquiry strengthen scholarship related to interprofessional competencies.
5. Prompt dialogue to identify goodness of fit between core competencies, practice, needs, and mandates (IPEC Expert Panel, 2011, p. 7).

In addition, the IPEC panel identified four domains of interprofessional collaborative practice (**TABLE 8-2**) and desired principles of the interprofessional competencies (**BOX 8-1**).

While the competency domains and specific competencies are general in nature and function, there is mutual agreement that they can position leaders of interprofessional teams to be successful. As teams accomplish project aims, mandates posed internally and externally will be met. However, project leaders must ensure that the team is aware of the realities inherent in any change and recognize that adaption is even more important than anticipation (Porter-O'Grady & Malloch, 2015).

TABLE 8-2 Interprofessional Collaborative Practice Domains

Competency Domain 1:	Values and Ethics for Interprofessional Practice
Competency Domain 2:	Roles and Responsibilities
Competency Domain 3:	Interprofessional Collaboration
Competency Domain 4:	Teams and Teamwork

Reproduced from Interprofessional Education Collaborative. (2016). *Core competencies for interprofessional collaborative practice: 2016 update.* Washington, DC: Interprofessional Education Collaborative.

BOX 8-1 Desired Principles of Interprofessional Competencies

- Patient centered
- Community and population oriented
- Relationship focused
- Process oriented
- Developmental learning activities, strategies, and behavioral assessments specific to the learner
- Integration across the continuum of learning
- Sensitive to systems and the applicability across all care settings
- Applicable across professions
- Stated in common and meaningful language across professions
- Outcome driven

(Reproduced from Association of American Medical Colleges (2011). *From Core Competencies for Interprofessional Collaborative Practice*, James L. Harris and Kathryn Ward-Presson; permission conveyed through Copyright Clearance Center, Inc.)

Managing any team, whether a clinical project team or a systems change team, requires leaders to keep in mind that the membership of the interprofessional team is a partnership among professionals, individuals, families, and communities. Team leadership and management are based on expertise and competencies that match the needs of the team. Decision-making and problem-solving are a shared responsibility, where information provided by patients and various disciplines is key for the success of any project endeavor (Simpson et al., 2001). While there is no assurance that a leader can manage a project team with 100% effectiveness, these ideas can turn the interprofessional project team into an energetic and productive enterprise.

▶ Measuring Interprofessional Project Leader Effectiveness

Researchers have argued that the effective leader is a key analyst of organizational function success or failure (Madanchian, Hussein, Noordin, & Taherdoost, 2017). This can easily be transferred when applied to measuring interprofessional project **team leader effectiveness**. Organizational learning requires that effectiveness be continuously assessed. This assists leaders to avoid pitfalls and strengthens their ability to manage interprofessional teams to be more effective.

Yukl (2008) argued that identifying leadership characteristics is paramount to improving leader and organizational effectiveness. Dhar and Mishra (2001) further advanced this idea by identifying outcomes used to assess leader effectiveness, which include: subordinate effectiveness, job satisfaction, commitment and performance, decision-making skills, and group performance. Identifying if expectations were met and changes improved outcomes is one strategy to assess interprofessional project team leader effectiveness.

▶ Summary

- Interprofessional team engagement is pivotal to quality, safe, and effective project outcomes.
- The five stages of team synergy include forming, storming, norming, performing, and adjourning.
- Using a common language that interprofessional team members understand and endorse will advance care delivery and continuous improvement.
- Coaching project teams requires leadership competencies as well as an understanding of interprofessional core competencies, the basic assumptions of team functioning, and guiding principles for productive and positive deliverables.
- As interprofessional team needs and competencies are identified, team leaders can capitalize on them to meet the project aim and create a productive enterprise.
- Measuring interprofessional project team leader effectiveness is pivotal to organizational learning for sustained growth and success.

Reflection Questions

1. For a member of an interprofessional project team, which characteristics are essential for efficient and effective management of the team toward accomplishing

the identified aim? How could you use the leader characteristics to lead a project team to successful outcomes?

2.   How can the use of a common language by project team members enhance or inhibit success?

3.   What are two primary needs of successful interprofessional teams? Discuss how you might use this information to meet various mandates in the current healthcare environment.

References

American Association of Colleges of Nursing. (2015). *Enhancing diversity in the workforce.* Retrieved from http://www.aacn.ache.edu/media-relations/fact-sheets/enhancing-diversity

Association of American Medical Colleges. (2011). *Core competencies for interprofessional collaborative practice.* Retrieved from https://nexusipe-resource-exchange.s3-us-west-2.amazonaws.com /IPEC_CoreCompetencies_2011.pdf

Begun, J., Zimmerman, B., & Dooley, K. (2003). Health care organizations as complex adaptive systems. In S. M. Mick & M. Wyttenback (Eds.), *Advances in health care organization theory.* San Francisco, CA: Jossey-Bass.

Chinn, P. (2008). *Peace and power.* Sudbury, MA: Jones and Bartlett Publishers.

Crisp, N. (2014). Mutual learning and reverse innovation: Where next? *Crisp Globalization and Health, 10*(14), 1–4.

Dhar, U., & Mishra, P. (2001). Leadership effectiveness: A study of constituent factors. *Journal of Management Research, 1*(4), 254.

Drinka, T., & Clark, P. (2000). *Healthcare teamwork: Interdisciplinary practice and teaching.* Westport, CT: Auburn House.

Dunevitz, B. (1997). Perspectives in ambulatory care: Collaboration—in a variety of ways—creates health care value. *Nursing Economics, 15*(4), 218–219.

Edmondson, A. C. (1999). Psychological safety and learning behavior in work teams. *Administrative Science Quarterly, 44,* 350–383.

Feldman, H. (2008). *Nursing leadership: A concise encyclopedia.* New York, NY: Springer.

Finkelman, A., & Kenner, C. (2010). *Professional nursing concepts: Competencies for quality leadership.* Sudbury, MA: Jones and Bartlett Publishers.

Gladwell, M. (2002). *The tipping point: How little things can make a big difference.* New York, NY: Back Bay Books/Little, Brown.

Goleman, D. (1998). *Working with emotional intelligence.* New York, NY: Bantam.

Goleman, D., Boyzatsis, R., & McKee, A. (2002). *Primal leadership: Realizing the power of emotional intelligence.* Boston, MA: Harvard Business School Press.

Hackman, J. T., & Wageman, R. (2005). A theory of team coaching. *Academy of Management Review, 30*(2), 269–287.

Hall, P., & Weaver, L. (2001). Interdisciplinary education and teamwork: A long and winding road. *Medical Education, 35,* 867–875.

Hanson, C. M., & Spross, J. A. (2009). Collaboration. In A. B. Hamric, J. A. Spross, & C. M. Hanson (Eds.), *Advanced practice nursing: An integrative approach* (4th ed., pp. 283–314). St. Louis, MO: Saunders Elsevier.

Hoying, C. (2017). Creating a business case for innovation. In S. Davidson, D. Weberg, T. Porter-O'Grady, & K. Malloch (Eds.), *Leadership for evidence-based innovation in nursing and health professions.* Burlington, MA: Jones & Bartlett Learning.

Institute of Medicine (IOM). (2001). *Crossing the quality chasm: A new health system for the 21st century.* Washington, DC: National Academies Press.

Interprofessional Education Collaborative (IPEC) Expert Panel. (2011). *Core competencies for interprofessional collaborative practice: Report of an expert panel.* Washington, DC: Interprofessional Education Collaborative.

Kennedy, B. (2016). Toward a just culture. *Nursing Management, 46*(6), 13–15.

Khatri, N., Brown, G. D., & Hicks, L. L. (2009). From a blame culture to a just culture in health care. *Health Care Management Review, 34*(4), 312–322.

Kotter, J. (1990). What leaders really do? *Harvard Business Review, 68,* 104.

Kouzes, J., & Pozner, B. (2007). *The leadership challenge*. San Francisco, CA: Wiley.

LaPorte, T. A. (2006). High reliability organizations: Unlikely, demanding and at risk. *Journal of Contingencies and Crisis Management, 4*(2), 60–71.

Leonard, M., Graham, S., & Bonacum, D. (2004). The human factor: The critical importance of effective teamwork and communication in providing safe care. *Quality and Safety in Health Care, 13*(Suppl. 1), 85–90.

Madanchian, M., Hussein, N., Noordin, F., & Taherdoost. H. (2017). Leadership effectiveness measurement and its effect on organizational outcomes. *Procedia Engineering, 181,* 1043–1048.

Martin, C. A., & Tulgan, B. (2006). *Managing generational mix: From urgency to opportunity*. Amherst, MA: HRD Press.

McCallin, A., & Bamford, A. (2007). Interdisciplinary teamwork: Is the influence of emotional intelligence fully appreciated? *Journal of Nursing Management, 15*(4), 386–391.

Naylor, M. (2012). Achieving high value transition care: The central role of nursing and its leadership. *Nursing Administration Quarterly, 36*(2), 115–126.

Patterson, K., Grenny, J., McMillian, R., & Switzler, A. (2002). *Crucial conversations: Tools for talking when stakes are high*. New York, NY: McGraw-Hill.

Porter-O'Grady, T., & Malloch, K. (2015). *Quantum leadership: Building better partnerships for sustainable health*. Burlington, MA: Jones & Bartlett Learning.

Scott-Cawiezell, J., Jones, K., Moore, L., & Vojir, C. (2004). Moving from a culture of blame to a just culture in the nursing home setting. *Nursing Forum, 41,* 133–140.

Simpson, G., Rabin, D., Schmitt, M., Taylor, P., Urban, S., & Ball, J. (2001). Interprofessional healthcare practice: Recommendations of the National Academies of Practice expert panel on healthcare in the 21st century. *Issues in Interdisciplinary Care, 3*(1), 5–19.

The Joint Commission. (2018). *National patient safety goals*. Retrieved from http://www.jointcommission .org/standards_information/npsgs.aspx

Tucker, A. L., Nembhard, I. M., & Edmondson, A. C. (2007). Implementing new practices: An empirical study of organizational learning in hospital intensive care units. *Management Science, 53,* 894–907.

Tuckman, B. W. (2001). Development sequence in small groups. *Group Facilitation: A Research and Applications Journal, 3,* 66–81.

World Health Organization (WHO). (2013). *Interprofessional collaborative practice in primary health care: Nursing and midwifery perspectives: Six case studies*. Geneva, Switzerland: Author.

Yukl, G. (2008). How leaders influence organizational effectiveness. *The Leadership Quarterly, 19*(6), 708–722.

Zaccagnini, M. E., & White, K. W. (2014). *The doctor of nursing practice essentials* (2nd ed.). Burlington, MA: Jones & Bartlett Learning.

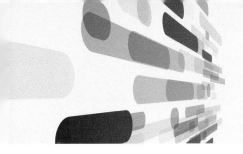

Case Exemplar

▶ **Case Study 1**

Transforming Care with Engaged Teams

Kathryn M. Ward-Presson

Background

Visionary leadership and interprofessional collaboration among all members of the healthcare leadership team are essential to improve patient care outcomes and meet Triple Aim objectives (Bisognano & Kenney, 2012). As a member of the "C suite," the chief nursing officer (CNO) routinely works with other executives such as the chief executive officer (CEO), chief of staff (COS), chief operating officer (COO), and chief financial officer (CFO) to identify organizational goals and determine clinical outcome measures and commensurate targets requiring priority focus. Goals and outcome measures identified should be consistent with those established by the facility's board of directors. Achieving goal attainment and the sustainability of improved patient outcomes depends on the selection of healthcare leadership team members who demonstrate effective project management and collegial problem-solving competencies (American Nurses Association, 2009; American Organization of Nurse Executives, 2007; Harris, Roussel, Walters, & Dearman, 2011).

Nursing's Role

The CNO and other nursing leaders hold pivotal roles that may positively influence the achievement of organizational quality improvement objectives. One example of that influence is seen with the successful execution of designated projects such as the implementation of clinical bundles to address patient outcome deficits. This is especially true when the organization's priority projects involve nurse-sensitive indicators such as rates of hospital-acquired pressure ulcers (HAPUs) and catheter-associated urinary tract infections (CAUTIs).

Facility Exemplar

The existence of higher-than-target (0%) HAPU and CAUTI rates in a large tertiary teaching and research healthcare facility provides an example highlighting strategies to improve these rates through the collaborative efforts of the facility's nursing staff and other members of the team. Creating effective senior and mid-level nursing leadership teams was essential to the nursing team's ability to work collegially with other disciplines and address unit-based (microsystem) and overall nursing (macrosystem) performance improvement (PI) initiatives. Any improvements achieved due to nursing interventions and partnerships with non-nurse colleagues also served to improve the organization's HAPU and CAUTI rates at the macrosystem level.

The CNO employed a variety of leadership assessment strategies (e.g., one-on-one sessions with each senior nursing leadership member, Strengths Finder 2.0 assessments [Rath, 2007], and small-group meetings) to determine senior nursing leadership team members' interests, strengths, challenges, and career goals. Each member's ability to work with all nursing staff and other disciplines was also examined. Individual professional development plans were implemented to assist with each member's growth and competency development. Similar strategies were adopted by senior nursing leaders when assessing and establishing development plans for their direct-report nurse managers.

Establishing a senior nurse leader role of "Performance Improvement and Practice" and identifying an individual to fill this position (someone who possessed the necessary advanced competencies in the application of evidence-based practice principles, data gathering, and analysis and staff engagement) was critical to providing oversight for nursing PI projects, a central repository for performance-related information, and the availability of a subject-matter expert to assist line staff with unit-based and global PI projects. The facility's existing nursing shared governance structure was also evaluated and strengthened to ensure staff participation reflective of all job categories throughout the continuum of care.

Nursing wound care specialists led the facility's wound care committee and engaged committee members from other disciplines (medicine, infection control, dietary, materials management, and pharmacy) to ensure the creation of an interprofessional forum to address needed improvements in policies, procedures, and processes related to the organization's pressure ulcer prevention program. The committee reviewed evidence-based HAPU bundles and led the rollout of the designated HAPU bundle on an organization-wide basis. This group also monitored HAPU bundle implementation progress and reported relevant outcomes data to the medical and nursing executive committees and the governing body. Similar interprofessional team creation and operational strategies were employed to address the facility's CAUTI bundle implementation and outcome monitoring/reporting project.

The facility's unit-based and overarching nursing PI committees and the Nurse Executive Council (NEC) were updated at least quarterly regarding progress toward meeting the 0% HAPU and CAUTI rate targets. Unit-based PI committees and NEC members evaluated the data, provided input regarding further opportunities to improve the efforts, and determined strategies that appeared to be more effective than others in decreasing either rate. Results and reports were presented visually in the form of graphs and run charts, and raw numbers with benchmarks were shared during small- and large-group meetings. Results were also posted on unit bulletin boards for all stakeholders to review. The information provided also included narrative discussions about the effectiveness of the interventions used. Summary information was incorporated in the organization's annual nursing report as well.

With the support of the organization's executive team, senior nursing leadership and the NEC developed another strategy to improve HAPU and CAUTI outcomes—the implementation of the clinical nurse leader (CNL) role. The CNL is a master's prepared nurse who possesses the competencies necessary to address the lateral integration of care delivery in collaboration with other healthcare disciplines and leads PI initiatives designed to improve patient care outcomes such as HAPU and CAUTI rates at the microsystem (unit) level (American Association of Colleges of

Nursing, 2007). A medical–surgical unit was selected as the target site for CNL role introduction, and a new graduate CNL (who had been a staff nurse on the designated unit) was selected. Although no statistically significant improvements were found within the first year of the CNL role implementation, clinical significance during the first year and zero unit HAPU and CAUTI rates were achieved 1 year after role implementation. Nursing leaders should consider the implementation of the CNL role as a strategy to foster interdisciplinary collaboration and clinical outcome improvements at the microsystem level. As noted previously, a healthcare facility's microsystem improvements may favorably impact macrosystem patient care outcomes and overall improvements to care delivery.

Reflection Questions

1. Consider a unit/organization and the Institute of Medicine's Triple Aim objectives. What are the priority clinical outcome improvement projects in the area? How and why were they selected?
2. Reflect upon an improvement conducted on a unit/organization. What was the outcome of the improvement project? How would you describe the effectiveness of those leading the project in ensuring collaboration among the key stakeholders? What did the leaders (formal and informal) do well to encourage team member engagement, and which suggestions do you have to improve full team-member participation?
3. Think about a unit or organization. How would the introduction of a different position, such as the clinical nurse leader, clinical educator, or clinical nurse specialist role, potentially impact team engagement and interprofessional collaboration to achieve project improvement success and positive outcomes? Which strategies would you use to introduce a new nursing role and ensure interprofessional collaboration and engagement?

References

American Association of Colleges of Nursing. (2007). *White paper on the role of the clinical nurse leader*. Retrieved from http://www.aacn.nche.edu/PublicationsandResources/WhitePapers/CNL

American Nurses Association. (2009). *Nursing administration scope and standards of practice*. Silver Spring, MD: Nursesbooks.org.

American Organization of Nurse Executives. (2007). *AONE guiding principles for the role of the nurse executive in patient safety*. Retrieved from http://www.aone.org/resources/role-nurse-executive-patient-safety.pdf

Bisognano, M., & Kenney, C. (2012). *Pursuing the triple aim*. San Francisco, CA: Jossey-Bass.

Harris, J. L., Roussel, L., Walters, S. E., & Dearman, C. (2011). *Project planning and management: A guide for CNLs, DNPs and nurse executives*. Sudbury, MA: Jones & Bartlett Learning.

Rath, T. (2007). *Strengths finders 2.0*. New York, NY: Gallup Press.

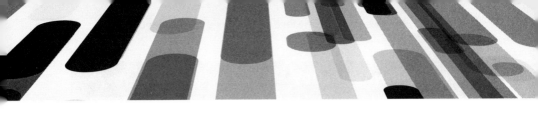

CHAPTER 9

Making the Case for a Project: Needs Assessment

Carolyn Thomas Jones
Linda Roussel

©Shuoshu/DigitalVision Vectors/Getty Images

PROFESSIONAL VALUES

Advocacy   Quality
Confidentiality

CORE COMPETENCIES

Advocacy   Design
Assessment   Development
Coordination   Stewardship
Data management   SWOT analysis

▶ Introduction

The identification of a need is the cornerstone of project planning when an organization is starting a new clinical program or a community is considering enhancing existing services. Unmet need motivates the formation of laws, policies, innovative practices, learning, treatment, and health service funding (Harrison, Young, Butow, & Solomon, 2013). Developing and conducting a needs assessment for a healthcare "project" is a project in itself. As described in Chapter 1, a project cycle evolves from initiation, to planning, to executing the project, to analysis and closure. A needs assessment requires determining the factors that may systematically identify specific need, the development of tools to measure those factors, carrying out the assessments using defined qualitative and quantitative methods, analysis of results, and closure. This then leads to next steps in project and/or program management. This chapter identifies what a **clinical needs assessment** evaluates, answers the question of why one completes a needs assessment, and outlines steps followed when completing the assessment.

The Institute of Medicine (IOM), in its pivotal report *Crossing the Quality Chasm* (2001), identified six specific aims and observable metrics required for the delivery of quality care (**FIGURE 9-1**). Each of these six aims can provide direction in developing a

SAFE	EFFECTIVE	EFFICIENT
Overall morbidity or mortality rates or % receiving care	How well EBP is followed *(ex. time diabetic pts receive all recommended care at each visit)*	Analysis of costs of care by patient, provider, organization & community

TIMELY	PATIENT-CENTERED	EQUITABLE
Waits and delays in receiving care, service, or results	Pt and family satisfaction	Differences in quality measures by race, gender, income and other factors

FIGURE 9-1 Six Aims and Metrics for Delivering Quality Care

Data from IOM. (2001). *Crossing the quality chasm: A new health system for the 21st century.*

needs assessment. A healthcare practitioner could apply several of the primary aims in one overarching project design, or just focus on a single element.

Consider the use of induced hypothermia (IH) care for patients brought to an emergency department (ED) because they have been resuscitated after sudden cardiac death. For emergency departments that have implemented this protocol, it is important to understand how well this program is operating and managing care by measuring several outcome factors based on the IOM's six aims:

- *Safe:* What percentage of patients who have experienced sudden cardiac death receive IH? What were the *mortality* rates or negative *morbidity* rates of this care?
- *Effective:* Is the protocol being carried out correctly? Are patients maintained in a hypothermic state for the correct amount of time? Are they rewarmed at the correct time and in an appropriate manner?
- *Efficient:* How has the ED budget been impacted by the launch of the IH program? How many staff are trained to deliver this care? How has this program affected staffing levels?
- *Timely:* Is the IH being performed rapidly enough (time from admission to ED to IH)?
- *Patient-centered:* What are the patient and family satisfaction scores, and how do they compare to scores for pre-IH care delivery for sudden cardiac death resuscitation admissions?
- *Equitable:* Are there disparities in how and to whom IH care is being delivered? Are patients with insurance treated differently than those who are uninsured?

These are skeletal examples of how to use the IOM's six aims and metrics for delivering quality care. Applying this rubric to project planning will aid in focusing the development of a robust needs assessment.

The World Health Organization (WHO, 2000) has defined a needs assessment as a tool for project and program planning. A needs assessment may be defined as a systematic review of the way things are and the way they should be (Rouda & Kusy, 1995). Wright, Williams, and Wilkinson (1998) stressed that health needs assessments are systematic measures that identify unmet needs of health and the system that can lead to actionable change.

Like any other research methodology, a needs assessment should be **transparent**, **reliable**, and **replicable**. Needs assessments are also dynamic processes. While the assessment may measure "need" or identify "unmet needs" at one point in time to establish a baseline reading, it also provides a means to identify positive or negative shifts, changes, and improvements. Needs assessments can use a combination of **qualitative** and **quantitative** data collection techniques. The steps and considerations for conducting a needs assessment are summarized in **BOX 9-1**.

The Community Tool Box (n.d.) is an excellent resource for completing a needs assessment survey. Specifically, questions that are important to consider are as follows:

1. What is the purpose (or goals) for doing this needs assessment survey? Drilling down on goals can help the team clarify reasons for doing the needs assessment and planning for the project. Other considerations include how the results may be used and how aligned the goals are with the overall purpose. Asking this question gives the team the opportunity to be clearer as a collective and have dialogue from all perspectives.

BOX 9-1 Steps to Planning a Needs Assessment

Step 1: Purpose
- What is known about the issue?
- What do you want to know?
- What will you do with the information?
- What are your biases?

Step 2: Population
- Who is being assessed: A community? A patient population? An institution? A department? A service? A treatment provider?
- What do stakeholders say about this population and approaches to measuring need? (Conduct focus groups or expert panels.)
- Will private health information be collected? How is confidentiality maintained?
- Will an informed consent form be needed?

Step 3: Method
- Will a survey be used?
- Will it be anonymous?
- Will it be observational?
- Will data collected be quantitative or qualitative?
- Which kind of sampling method will be used?

Step 4: Instrument
- Are reliable and valid tools being used?
- Will new tools be developed?
- Are questions or queries clearly stated and without bias?
- How will responses be recorded or measured?
- How easy is it to use the instrument?
- Does it include culturally competent language?
- Can results be easily summarized and analyzed?
- Will institutional review board (IRB) review and approval be required? Which type?

Step 5: Data Collection
- Is there a data management system for collecting and organizing data?
- A data dictionary?
- Key data categories?
- Calculation methods?
- Missing or incomplete data?

Step 6: Analyses
- What are results?
- What are the assessment's limitations?

Step 7: Use the Results
- Short-term and long-term goals
- Resource allocation
- Summarized findings
- Dissemination plans

2. Is the timing right for the needs assessment? The team questions the preparation needed to do the work with high-quality effort. It is important that timing and resources are in tandem and that resources are available. The team needs to be assured that the timing necessary to do the needs assessment survey from start to finish has been thought through at every step.

3. Has the team considered the number of individuals who need to be involved in taking the needs assessment survey? Has the team considered the kinds of people (consumers, stakeholders) who will offer the most relevant information to inform decisions about the overall purpose of the project? Following the purpose (goals) and timing, individuals and groups germane to the needs assessment can be asked to offer insights, feedback, and perspectives that will provide a more robust conceptualization of the need and project.

4. Who (on the team) is best suited to ask the questions (needs assessment survey/interview)? Considering the community and insider perspective, individuals "closest" to the individuals who will be impacted by the project would be best suited to connect the purpose with the plan.

In 2000, WHO identified three evaluation components that should be considered and/ or adopted in the needs assessment process for healthcare services for a given population:

■   Capacity of services in relation to prevalence and incidence of a syndrome or disease in a specific area
■   Mix of services required or desired for a syndrome or disease
■   Coordination of services in a healthcare delivery system whereby entry, transition, and follow-up occur and are standard practice (WHO 2000)

▶ Purpose of Needs Assessment

When assessing needs and capacity within an organization, a SWOT analysis is often used. This assessment identifies the strengths, weaknesses, opportunities, and threats impacting an organization at a point in time. SWOT analyses have been used for assessing needs and performing strategic planning in healthcare organizations (van Wijngaarden, Scholten, & van Wijk, 2012). They unpack the dichotomies between external developments (opportunities or threats) and internal capabilities (strengths and weaknesses). A proposed model for SWOT analysis includes a three-pronged approach for its implementation:

■   Stakeholder expectations: demands and standards
■   Contextual factors: trends and network developments
■   Resources: capabilities, people, finance, and means

The goals for a project needs assessment should be clearly identified and should provide a guide for data collection. The basic components of a needs assessment address the differences between what is known about the idea and what is still unknown. A tenet for all scholarly work, including needs assessment, is "If you do not need to know the answer, then do not ask the question." Therefore, all known and unknown elements and their impact must be assessed to determine their fit with the project. The ultimate goal of any project is to produce usable results that will positively impact functions and deliverables within the organization. If not, then one must ask, "Why did you do it?"

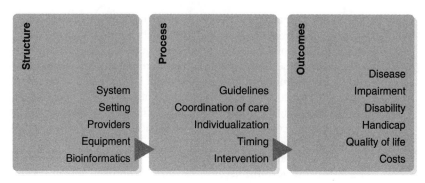

FIGURE 9-2 Donabedian Model: Structure, Process, and Outcomes

An important element in identification of purpose and need is the identification of biases within the project team, the stakeholders, and the organization as a whole. The needs assessment data can also serve as a guide to project financial impact, justify the allocation of funding by the funding source, and provide support for the **business case**. Business cases are guided by data that validate inefficiencies, the unpredictable nature of organizations, occupational differences, and interdependencies within and across systems.

Another method of assessing quality-associated care and the planning of new projects is to apply the semi-qualitative method developed by Donabedian (1998). This approach is based on three key components: structure, process, and outcomes. Each of these components has direct influence on the others, in a sequential fashion. *Structure* refers to the healthcare setting: personnel (staff expertise), material resources (e.g., electronic health records), and organizational structure (hospital, clinic). *Process* refers to what is done. *Outcomes* refers to health outcomes. Assembling data into these three "buckets" (**FIGURE 9-2**) can assist in better understanding the next steps in identifying key needs and proposed project plans for evolving improvements.

▶ Population

The population of interest must be described, whether the project is focused on an organization, a patient population, or a community. The purpose of the project will guide identification of the population.

Once the population is identified, the project leader and/or team must determine the stakeholders' perception of the problem that the project is designed to address. Project team members must collect information from all **stakeholders** to facilitate an effective problem resolution. Stakeholders may include the following groups: (1) patients or those experiencing the need, (2) health and human services providers, (3) government officials, (4) influential people, (5) people whose jobs are impacted by the proposed actions that would result from the assessment, (6) community activists, and (7) affected local businesses.

Population assessment methods can include expert panels, focus groups, surveys, and interviews, among others. The method selected should fit both the population and the project. During this assessment phase, project team members should also determine the level of data that will be collected. For example, if private health information is

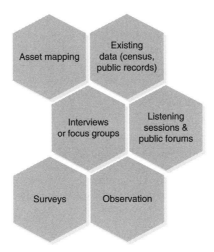

FIGURE 9-3 Sources and Methods for Measuring Community Needs

needed to carry out the project and produce a viable product, then the project team must determine how that information will be collected, protected, stored, and used.

Questions related to maintenance of confidentiality, anonymity, and informed consent must be considered. Will data be reported, individually or in aggregate format? How will the research/project team assure security of all information? Inherent in these considerations is "goodness of fit": Do the data fit the purposes of the project, and will they yield the desired results? These and other questions provide much context for the project and are also considerations when measuring community needs, as illustrated in **FIGURE 9-3**.

Recruiting stakeholder participants requires preplanning. It is not uncommon to use more than one method to contact existing and potential stakeholders:

- Social media postings
- Random selection (from telephone directories)
- Mail or email
- Observation of behavior
- Stopping people in public places
- Posters/fliers in public places
- Radio/TV/newspaper advertisement
- Community group outreach
- Personal networking
- Internet surveys (direct to database)

▶ Methods and Instruments

Project personnel should select the method of data collection and either locate or develop instruments that will best fit the project and the methods. Surveys, for example, are a popular method of gathering information from larger groups. When developing survey questions, it is important to be concise and clear. Questions that fall into categorical (or nominal) level categories should be separated from those that fall in ordinal levels.

An example of a nominal-level question is:

Categorize your highest educational level:

    a.   Some high school
    b.   High school graduate/GED
    c.   Some college
    d.   College graduate
    e.   Post-baccalaureate

An example of an ordinal-level question would be:

Protected learning time for emergency department staff members should be increased to 1 hour per month:

    a.   Strongly agree
    b.   Agree
    c.   Disagree
    d.   Strongly disagree

These types of questions can be incorporated into surveys, questionnaires, and interviews.

Other considerations related to methods of data collection include determining whether the data are best captured through a qualitative or quantitative approach. The sampling method to be used is another important component. Samples must be representative of the population and must be sufficient in number to support the findings.

In any project, there is always the possibility of uncovering potential problems in an organization at the micro-, meso-, or macrolevel when one is completing a needs assessment. Loo (2003) proposed two methods that organizations may consider using when such problems or issues are identified: an issues analysis chart and an issues impact assessment. An issues analysis chart assists in describing the problem, its impact, and required actions. It complements an issues impact assessment by identifying how the problem(s) may become a barrier to initiating the project and which negative impacts may arise if the problems occur as the project is being completed.

Oliva and Rockart (1997) suggested three other considerations to be taken into account when an organization is conducting a clinical needs assessment: (1) inter-program complementarities, (2) inter-program competition, and (3) interactions among and between programs and services. First, whether or not a project or program was successfully implemented and sustained, organizations must assess how previous projects and programs might have benefited the current endeavor. It is important to determine if tools can be used again or modified for future use. Moreover, if shifts in knowledge, organizational culture, performance, or attitudes occur, those shifts should be measured. Second, organizations should assess the benefits or challenges associated with inter-program competition. Conflicts across programs or competitive programs can become barriers rather than facilitators of the organization's mission, vision, and purpose. Barriers can result in fragmented roles and performance outcomes and ultimately erode employee motivation, resulting in a domino effect of mounting cynicism and deterioration of management's leadership. Finally, organizations must consider the interactions within and between programs and services and examine each program's contributions to the overall success of each unit, the broader organization, and quality of care that will follow.

The IOM (1999) suggests that problems associated with quality of care can be organized into the three categories illustrated in **FIGURE 9-4**. Underuse, overuse, and

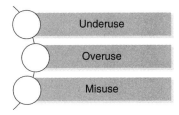

FIGURE 9-4 Three Categories for Healthcare Quality

misuse may stem from clinical guidelines, policies, equipment, staffing, informatics, authority, funding sources, and many other elements that are at play in structuring and managing a healthcare facility in acute care, long-term care, ambulatory care, or community care.

An example of underuse may occur with electronic medical record data. Nurses and staff who input data into electronic medical records spend a tremendous amount of time on this task. Some of those data are redundant, however; other data are not accessed or used on a routine basis to deliver care. As a consequence, the time spent documenting in the electronic record may not correspond directly to those data's ultimate utility.

Another example is "work-arounds." Nurses often use work-arounds to facilitate the daily activities involved in performing their jobs. For example, some may employ personal mobile devices that aid in getting the job done but which may be a violation of institutional policy and could jeopardize patient privacy. Such work-arounds may represent overuse or misuse issues that impact quality performance and care.

Innovative and creative problem solving can lead to improvements in care delivery; however, it is important to collect data on the utility and risks/benefits of such initiatives. In doing so, it can be useful to consider the underuse, overuse, and misuse issues that are observable and measurable in the organization. Closing gaps in those areas can have a strong positive impact on both quality care and cost savings. The needs assessment is a first step toward planning a project that can address those gaps.

▶ Human Subject Protections and Institutional Review Board Requirements

The protection of human subjects and adherence to research regulations require an understanding of the subtle differences between quality improvement activities and clinical research. It is especially important to determine if there is a need for informed consent, including the requirement for **institutional review board (IRB)** review and approval. Some may question whether IRB approval is necessary when quality improvement processes and quality assessments are the foci. That argument goes like this: "Since the IRB is predominantly focused on the ethical conduct of research, why should quality improvement projects be reviewed by the IRB? After all, quality improvement is not research."

The response to this argument is that IRB approvals may be necessary for both patient welfare and institutional regulatory adherence. Patients are the focus of quality improvement, process improvement, and research projects, and therefore their rights

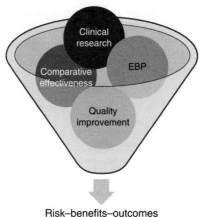

Risk–benefits–outcomes

FIGURE 9-5 Types of Healthcare "Research"

must be protected (Speers, 2008). Similarly, **community needs assessments** can impact individuals and populations; thus, protection is warranted for communities as well. Moreover, failure to obtain IRB approval can lead to institutional fines and disqualification of the research by federal authorities.

Quality improvement and clinical research share similar aims and are often intermingled. As a consequence, it is sometimes difficult to distinguish between a quality improvement effort and a research effort. Because regulations and bioethical guidelines have evolved, it is important to rely on current requirements when addressing this issue, rather than on comments and opinions of persons who may not currently be knowledgeable about these requirements. When in doubt, ask the IRB. In each case (i.e., a quality improvement effort and a research effort), the project leader may formulate a hypothesis (research question or problem statement), determine risks and benefits, and define methodology and outcomes measures. If IRB approval is required, final official approval must be in place prior to any data collection. The type of IRB approval needed will depend on the organization or institutional policies and federal regulations.

Assessments can sometimes cross into the gray zone of "research" based on their level of intensity. For instance, along the continuum between research and direct patient care are various levels of research assessments that contribute to our understanding of quality improvement, evidence-based practice, comparative effectiveness, and clinical research. Examples of the various types of healthcare research are illustrated in **FIGURE 9-5**. This topic is covered in more detail in Chapter 6: The Institutional Review Board Process.

▶ Instruments

The **validity** (Does the instrument measure what it is designed to measure?) and **reliability** (Does the instrument measure the concepts/constructs consistently in different settings, populations, or projects?) of an instrument are integral in determining the usefulness of the project outcomes. If existing tools are available that fit the project, the project team must determine the validity and reliability of those instruments. Traditionally, the validity and reliability of an instrument are described in the original and subsequent research studies that were used to establish them.

If instruments exist but must be altered, the project team must contact the author(s) of the tool and seek permission to use and modify it. Once modified, the instrument must be subjected to procedures to establish the validity and reliability of the modified sections.

If an instrument does not exist that will effectively measure the concepts and constructs of the project, then the researcher or project team may develop a new instrument for use with the project. All researcher- or project team–developed instruments must have their validity and reliability established. Most research texts provide a clear description of the processes and procedures involved in establishing validity and reliability. The reader is encouraged to review such a text for further discussion of this topic.

Instruments must be applicable to the project, expedient, and easy to use. These characteristics are essential not only in collecting data but also in collating, analyzing, and summarizing the data and disseminating the findings.

▶ Data Collection

Whether the research or project is large or small, a data management system for collecting and organizing data will be helpful. Data management systems can be quite simple. All that is needed is a mechanism to track the sample involved in the project with regard to where members of the sample are in the process. All team members can use this data management system to determine where each participant is with regard to stage of recruitment, informed consent, data collection, and other stages and can readily see which data points remain to be collected. The grid shown in **FIGURE 9-6** is a simple method of managing key data categories.

A data dictionary or glossary is another useful tool, especially if different members of the team are involved with collecting, categorizing, and entering data. Internal consistency of team usage will facilitate "clean" data collection and entry. Further, consistency in data collection will greatly ease data retrieval and analysis.

The final steps in data collection are determining consistent calculation methods and retrieving missing or incomplete data. Preliminary planning as to how partial and incomplete responses will be incorporated in the findings will assist with these processes.

Participant ID number	Informed consent	Instrument 1	Instrument 2	Data input complete
	Date out/received	Date out/received	Date out/received	

FIGURE 9-6 Data Collection Grid

▶ Analysis and Use of Findings

Once the data have been collected, they must be analyzed and applied within the organization/system. Any findings must be clearly described and linked back to the original short- and long-term goals and objectives of the project.

Once findings are published, at least internally, resource allocation processes for full implementation can begin. Dissemination of findings to a broader audience will be directly linked to organizational goals and objectives. At this point, the current study and project are considered to have ended, and another problem identification and needs assessment cycle begins.

▶ Summary

- Needs are the cornerstones for project planning.
- Clinical needs and community assessments provide the rationale and support for the project's business case.
- A series of steps is followed when completing a clinical needs assessment and a community needs assessment.
- A variety of tools can assist the project team when completing a needs assessment.
- Institutional review board approval may be required for projects, especially when the data will be disseminated beyond the organization. Approval is also suggested for internal system data dissemination in support of human-subjects protection.

Reflection Questions

1. Which elements are part of successful clinical needs assessment?
2. How are community needs assessments similar or different?
3. What should be considered before beginning the IRB approval process?
4. Conduct a CINAHL (Cumulative Index of Nursing and Allied Health Literature) search for the term "health needs assessment." Note the variety of needs assessments published. Focus your search on needs assessments in a population of interest to you. Begin to formulate best approaches for conducting a needs assessment for that population.

Learning Activities

Using Box 9-1 (Steps to Planning a Needs Assessment Outline), describe ways this tool provides foundational information in planning a project.

The Donabedian model (structure, process, outcome) can provide a framework for any project. Using the model, describe each concept in your current project.

References

Community Tool Box (n.d.). *Conducting needs assessment surveys, Section 7, Chapter 3*. Retrieved from https://ctb.ku.edu/en/table-of-contents/assessment/assessing-community-needs-and-resources /conducting-needs-assessment-surveys/main

Donabedian, A. (1988). The quality of care. How can it be assessed? *Journal of the American Medical Association, 269*(12), 1743–1748.

Harrison, J. D., Young, J. M., Butow, P. N., & Solomon, M. J. (2013). Needs in healthcare: What beast is that? *International Journal of Health Services, 43*(3), 567–585.

Institute of Medicine (IOM). (1999). *To err is human.* Washington DC: National Academies Press. Retrieved from http://nationalacademies.org/hmd/reports/1999/to-err-is-human-building-a-safer-health-system.aspx?_ga=2.48614627.439078995.1520992418-1302790904.1520992418

Institute of Medicine (IOM). (2001). *Crossing the quality chasm: A new health system for the 21st century.* Washington, DC: National Academies Press. Retrieved from http://nationalacademies.org/hmd/reports/2001/crossing-the-quality-chasm-a-new-health-system-for-the-21st-century.aspx?_ga=2.52343660.439078995.1520992418-1302790904.1520992418

Loo, R. (2003). Project management: A core competency for professional nurses and nursemanagers. *Journal of Nurses in Staff Development, 19*(4), 187–193.

Oliva, R., & Rockart, S. (1997). *Dynamics of multiple improvement efforts: The program life cycle model.* Retrieved from http://www.systemdynamics.org/conferences/1997/paper166.htm

Rouda, R. H., & Kusy, M. E. (1995). *Needs assessment: The first step.* Retrieved from http://alumnus.caltech.edu/-rouda/T2_NA.html

Speers, M. A. (2008). Editorial: Quality improvement: Research or non-research? AAHRPP perspective. *Association for the Accreditation of Human Research Protection Programs, Advance, 5*(2), 1–2.

Van Wijngaarden, J. D. H., Scholten, G. R. M., & van Wijk, K. P. (2012). Strategic analyses for healthcare organizations: The suitability of the SWOT-analysis. *International Journal of Health Planning and Management, 27*, 34–49.

World Health Organization (WHO). (2000). *Needs assessment: Workbook 3.* Retrieved from http://whqlibdoc.who.int/hq/2000/WHO_MSD_MSB_00.2d.pdf

Wright, J., Williams, R., & Wilkinson, J. R. (1998). Development and importance of health needs assessment. *British Medical Journal, 316*(7140), 1310–1313.

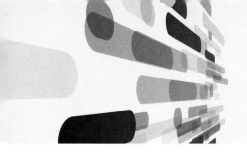

Case Exemplars

Applications for Project Planning and Management in Antimicrobial Stewardship

Dr. Carolynn Jones

Core elements and guidelines for a hospital-based antimicrobial stewardship (AMS) program have been described by the Centers for Disease Control and Prevention (CDC, 2014). The impact of antibiotic resistance continues to rank as one of the rising unmet medical needs. "The CDC estimates that more than two million people are infected with antibiotic resistant organisms in approximately 23,000 deaths annually" (p. 3). Moreover, antibiotic prescribing is inappropriate in 20% to 50% of such prescriptions and is contributing to the rising levels of resistance (**FIGURE 9-7**).

While the primary goal of AMS programs is to improve patient care and public health, a by-product of implementing and tracking these measures is huge financial savings to institutions and the healthcare enterprise. The aim is to use the correct agent, correct dose, and appropriate duration of dosing for desired outcomes in cure or prevention, minimization of toxicity, and prevention of development of resistant organisms. Institutional costs of implementing an antimicrobial resistance program (whether in an inpatient or ambulatory setting) are minimal compared to the resulting

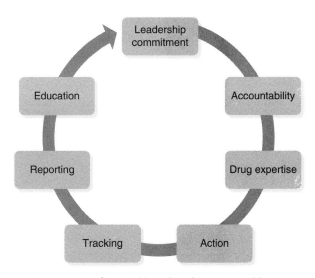

FIGURE 9-7 Seven Components of Hospital-based Antibiotic Stewardship Programs

health and financial savings. Building and maintaining sustainability in managing an AMS program is, therefore, an essential challenge for healthcare organizations.

Supporting a business case for ongoing measures requires continuous assessment of need, impact, and resource requirements. Manning (2014) discusses the urgent need for nurse practitioners (NPs) to lead AMS programs in ambulatory care settings and estimates that NPs in those settings write an average 19 prescriptions per day, many of which are for antibiotics. Bedside nurses and infection control nurses have an increasing role in every aspect of AMS.

Project planning and management of a variety of facets of AMS are ripe for advanced practice nurse involvement, whether as a clinician, a nurse executive, or a program manager. After developing a focused approach for problem identification in AMS, the NP should consider how to assess needs from clinical, pharmaceutical, financial, and resource perspectives. A key challenge in such a huge undertaking will be to focus attention on one population, specific organisms, or specific settings, for instance, so as to affect that critical issue positively and bring the project to fruition. Electronic medical record searches based on ICD and CPT coding and use of resources like the Premier Database (www.premierinc.com) are informatics-based approaches that can streamline assessment mechanisms to build a case for project planning and management and offer methods of tracking outcomes.

▶ Case Study 1

Project Planning Opportunities Using Case Findings

Dr. Carolynn Jones

A 58-year-old woman was driven to a community hospital emergency department (ED) at 2:30 a.m. by her 84-year-old mother, with complaints of severe epigastric abdominal pain that is reported to be a "15" on a 10-point pain scale. The pain is "constant, but comes in intense waves." The patient, who is a nurse, states, "This is not a typical stomach issue like virus or flu. Something is wrong. I am worried I have some sort of an acute abdomen. Something is not right."

On assessment, the patient has low-grade fever, a heart rate of 110, and a normal blood pressure (110/60 mm Hg); she appears to be in distress. Beyond vital signs, no other physical assessment is performed. The patient denies vomiting and diarrhea. Medical history reveals current medications: Prilosec (for chronic heartburn secondary to hiatal hernia), Zocor, and Ramipril (for mild hypertension).

Four weeks prior, the patient had begun treatment with azithromycin for culture-proven *Mycoplasma* pneumonia at a local freestanding acute care facility. Because her symptoms persisted after 10 days, she was prescribed a course of levofloxacin; however, no second culture was obtained. She was sent for an abdominal computed tomography (CT) scan with contrast within 3 hours of arrival and afterward began vomiting. The CT scan was negative. The patient was sent home with a probable diagnosis of "stomach bug" and was given a prescription for ondansetron and pain medication. Once home, the patient began to have diarrhea and continued to vomit. Her stomach pain remained extreme, and she was unable to sleep, maintaining a stressed, guarded position. She called a neighbor who was a gastroenterologist, who suggested she go to a different ED immediately.

After presentation to the ED, the patient was admitted to a triage room. Because of her weakened state, extreme pain, and light-headedness, an electrocardiogram (EKG) was performed, which was negative for signs of cardiac ischemia. An abdominal ultrasound was performed and was negative. She was again sent home with a tentative diagnosis of "stomach flu." Her nausea and vomiting persisted, however, and she reported having diarrhea.

On day 4, she pulled some strings and obtained an infectious disease consultation at a local academic medical center outpatient clinic, bringing a stool sample. Because she was taking a proton-pump inhibitor (Prilosec) and had prior antibiotic exposure, the patient was concerned that her continued stomach pain and issues were related to *Clostridium difficile* infection, a condition in which bacteria overgrowth releases toxins that attack the lining of the intestines; it can lead to peritonitis and death after structural ruptures. The infectious disease physician thought the diagnosis was possible but not probable, given the patient's age and lack of apparent autoimmune disorder. He prescribed metronidazole to be taken for 2 weeks but told her to hold off filling the prescription until stool culture results were confirmatory.

After 3 days, the patient was called and told to begin taking Flagyl—her stool cultures were positive for *C. difficile*. If her symptoms resolved, the patient was to commence high-dose probiotic therapy. If her symptoms did not resolve, she was eligible to consider enrollment in a study protocol using fecal microbiota transplant (FMT). Ultimately, her symptoms subsided with the single 14-day course of metronidazole.

Nursing Implications

C. difficile infections affects 500,000 Americans each year, mostly in hospitals and long-term facilities; however, as many as 36% of those cases are community acquired. Risk factors in community-acquired cases include antibiotic use, use of proton-pump inhibitors, and lung infections.

Case Study Issues

Consider opportunities for project planning and management for community-acquired *C. difficile* infections based on this case study.

1. The patient's medical history revealed risk factors for *C. difficile* infection.
2. The second round of antibiotics for mycoplasma pneumonia may have been unnecessary.
3. Medical staff at two local hospital EDs demonstrated lack of knowledge about *C. difficile*.
4. Stool cultures were not obtained at either ED visit.
5. The patient's persistence in seeking care, intuition about her condition, and use of influence to obtain an infectious disease consultation resulted in correct assessment and diagnosis; most patients lack this knowledge and self-advocacy and require advocacy on their behalf by healthcare practitioners.
6. The infectious disease physician followed an AMS program by awaiting culture results before commencing Flagyl therapy.
7. Probiotic therapy is essential for restructuring normal bacterial flora in the gut.
8. The highly contagious *C. difficile* infection requires home-based measures to reduce reinfection or spread of infection to elderly or otherwise compromised persons. All underwear and towels must be washed in hot water with bleach. All surfaces must be washed down frequently with bleach. Avoid sharing bathrooms, if possible. Strict hand washing should be observed.

▶ Case Study 2

Using Tools to Meet Patient Needs

Dr. Carolynn Jones

Intensive care nursing is fraught with daily challenges in addressing the clinical needs of patients with high acuity and managing diagnostic, pharmaceutical, and technological elements of care. Often lacking is attention to the basic oral care needs of patients. Consider the impact of poor oral hygiene in critically ill populations and preventable morbidity outcomes. Translate those outcomes into the financial burden imposed on insured persons, insurers, and the healthcare system.

Case Study Issues

Review a study published by Yildiz, Durna, and Akin (2013) that assessed the unmet medical needs (oral mucous membranes of intensive care unit patients) and the personal and treatment-related variables that impacted the delivery of oral care.

1. Discover the tools used to measure needs and outcomes. How were those data analyzed and presented?
2. What might be the next steps in project planning and management based on these findings?
3. Which other studies in oral care contribute to these findings?
4. Which treatment guidelines exist to support program planning?

▶ Case Study 3

Using a Mixed-Methods Approach to Assess Chronic Disease Needs in Low-Resource Countries

Dr. Carolynn Jones

The World Health Organization (2001, p. 1) defines community health needs assessment as a process that "describes the state of health of local people; enables the identification of major risk factors and causes of ill health; and enables the identification of actions needed to address these." Studies of chronic disease epidemiology and practices in low-resource countries are limited. To provide care in these settings requires an understanding of disease rates and the facilitators of and barriers to appropriate management and patient healthcare educational needs. Effecting change in these settings requires a stakeholder approach to best identify future healthcare and research needs.

Case Study Issues

Review a published study by Dekker, Amick, Scholcoff, and Doobay-Persaud (2017) that used a mixed-methods approach to determine chronic disease care gaps for diabetes mellitus and hypertension among rural populations in the district of Toledo, Belize.

1. How did this study use a stakeholder approach to identifying gaps?
2. Characterize the healthcare system and patient population under study.
3. The study used a mixed-methods approach. What were the multi-tiered levels of assessment in this study? Which were quantitative and which were qualitative?
4. What gaps were identified that could lead to future research and care?
5. Generate a research question that might evolve from these study results.
6. Compare and contrast this study and other needs assessments performed in low-resource countries for chronic disease management and resources.

References

Centers for Disease Control and Prevention (CDC). (2014). *Core elements of hospital antibiotic stewardship programs*. Atlanta, GA: U.S. Department of Health and Human Services. Retrieved from http://www.cdc.gov/getsmart/healthcare/implementation/core-elements.html

Dekker A. M., Amick A. E., Scholcoff C., & Doobay-Persaud A. (2017). A mixed-methods needs assessment of adult diabetes mellitus (type II) and hypertension care in Toledo, Belize. *BMC Health Services Research, 17*(1), 171. http://doi.org.proxy.lib.ohio-state.edu/10.1186/s12913-017-2075-9

Manning, M. L. (2014). The urgent need for nurse practitioners to lead antimicrobial stewardship in ambulatory health care [Editorial]. *Journal of the American Association of Nurse Practitioners, 26*, 411–413.

World Health Organization. (2001). *Community health needs assessment: An introductory guide for the family health nurse in Europe*. Retrieved from http://www.euro.who.int/__data/assets/pdf_file/0018/102249/E73494.pdf

Yildiz, M., Durna, Z., & Akin, S. (2013). Assessment of oral care needs of patients treated at the intensive care unit. *Journal of Clinical Nursing, 22*, 2734–2747.

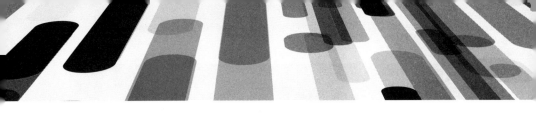

CHAPTER 10

Using Findings from the Clinical Needs Assessment to Develop, Implement, and Manage Sustainable Projects

Linda Roussel
Shea Polancich
Murielle S. Beene

KEY TERMS

Agility   Metrics
Evidence

ROLES

Decision maker   Leader
Implementation project manager   Risk anticipator

PROFESSIONAL VALUES

Accountability   Evidence-based
Commitment

CORE COMPETENCIES

Assessment   Management
Leadership

▶ Introduction

Developing, implementing, and managing a project can be a challenging experience, from moving the original idea to planning, carrying out the project, studying the results, and acting on outcomes. Put simply, these steps put the planned work into an actionable framework. Only an estimated 37% of projects are successful (Krigsman, 2011)—a low rate attributed to the often-limited time and resources spent to determine the project's overall value to the system. Understanding how to use a value equation and value proposition statement is essential to any possible success. Without a deep dive into understanding the organization's overall mission and goal, a project may squander resources, deliver poor financial returns, create substandard operating processes, compromise products and services to patients, and reduce stakeholders' returns. Despite improved project management methodologies, software development methodologies, and training in those methodologies, there has not been an appreciable increase in the success rate for project implementation over the past 20 years (Phelan & Stockwell, 2014).

The importance of using findings from a needs assessment to inform the developing, planning, and implementing phases of a project cannot be understated. The role of the implementation project manager is essential to this accomplishment, particularly from an interprofessional, collaborative perspective. When managing projects, it is important to have a leader who possesses strong communication skills, is results oriented, understands organizational dynamics, and is committed to corporate values. A close and mutually reinforcing (supportive) relationship exists between developing, planning, implementing, and monitoring. This chapter discusses the value of collaboration in a project's life cycle and the role of the implementation project manager. A description of a systems change model is provided as an example that can assist readers in answering key questions that support project implementation and sustainability in practice settings.

▶ Project Life Cycle: Role of the Clinical Needs Assessment

The project life cycle consists of four phases: initiation, planning, execution, and evaluation (Gido & Clements, 2015).

In the *initiation* phase of the project life cycle, the scope, purpose, objectives, resources, deliverables, timescales, and structure of the project are defined. These definitions are guided by the results of a clinical needs assessment. A clinical needs assessment considers information (data) from a variety of sources. These data are quantified—for example, length of stay, cost of a day in the intensive care unit, and infection rates. Qualitative data obtained through interviews, focus groups, and observations can add further depth to the needs assessment. A microsystem analysis using the five P's (purpose, population, processes, patterns, and providers) is a helpful assessment tool for obtaining internal data related to the organization and the larger system. With a thorough microsystem analysis, gaps can be identified—for example, between benchmarks and actual infection and falls rates—and further drilled down through a root cause analysis (RCA) and a failure mode effects analysis (FMEA):

■ RCA gets at the core of a complication or problem and considers all aspects of why a particular work process or patient care intervention has not worked as intended, perhaps leading to a fatal event. This type of analysis is generally done after the adverse advent.

■ FMEA is a proactive risk mitigation tool that identifies areas of potential failure and considers the severity and probability that a failure will occur. Hazard scores are then assigned based on the severity and frequency of the misstep (failed action) in the process.

RCA and FMEA are tools and processes that give the project team direction when considering the level of information needed to improve the overall process. Their results, which are considered internal data, are essential in determining the need to move forward to improve quality of work and care delivery. Internal data provide the necessary **evidence** and often baseline information for developing a business case, which often includes solutions and a cost-benefit analysis for each possible action for improvement. The feasibility of any one intervention (or a bundle of actions) should be thoroughly considered to ensure that the solution is realistic and has an acceptable level of risk. A project team is chartered to assure that all aspects of the initial plan (the business case) have been thoughtfully considered and to collectively step through the process to assure consensus and investment in the project plan's success (Gido & Clements, 2015).

Internal data collection can also include the use of a variety of assessment tools. For example, the Institute for Healthcare Improvement (IHI, 2017) provides an

Improvement Capability Self-Assessment Tool created to help organizations in assessing their capability in six key areas that support improvement:

- Leadership for Improvement
- Results
- Resources
- Workforce and Human Resources
- Data Infrastructure and Management
- Improvement Knowledge and Competence

The tool describes levels of capability and is intended as a baseline indication of the improvement capability of a healthcare system in a number of domains associated with overall improvement success. The levels include Just Beginning, Developing, Making Progress, Significance Impact, and Exemplary. For example, Leadership for Improvement, at a Just Beginning level, might be described as leadership not coordinated across departments or services with very little, if any, learning from improvement activities shared across the healthcare system. This level could serve as a baseline when you begin this assessment. Moving from Just Beginning to Exemplary would indicate progress and an ongoing measure of improvement. The information on the tool can be confidential, and the more honest the assessment, the greater the opportunities that the initiatives selected will be aligned with current ability and probability of success. This tool can be used by hospital leaders and staff in a number of ways, including stimulating discussion about areas of strength and weakness, to better understand current improvement capability, and to reflect on and evaluate specific improvement efforts (IHI, 2017).

Collecting internal data is important in the *planning* phase, which includes a detailed project plan created and monitored by the project manager and referred to throughout the life of the project. The monitoring aspect includes examining results such as costs and quality of expected outcomes. Particular aspects of the project plan include specific information on resources (staffing, equipment, supplies), finances (cost-benefit analysis, return on investment), quality (benchmarks, dashboard, key indicators for effective outcomes), risks (what could go wrong and how to mitigate or minimize such events), and deliverables (executive summary, manuscript, presentations). It is important to know what to expect to deliver before the team goes too far into implementing the plan (taking action). Accountability for particular deliverables must be established early on in the planning phase to assure that dissemination of results and sustainability are as important as implementing and evaluating the overall results (Gido & Clements, 2015).

Execution involves staying on task when implementing the action plan. The project manager and the team consider monitoring of time (tracking and recording time spent on the various aspects of the plan), cost (under/over budget), quality (indicators, outcomes), change (was there enough preparation in readying the environment for the change?), risks (were strategies taken to minimize risk and eliminate barriers?), buy-in (is there acceptance of the intervention strategies taken?), and communication (does information flow freely; is there transparency in how the project is going?). A communication plan is important to ensuring that all stakeholders are kept apprised of the actions taken, any complications or risks mitigated, and success (or failure) in realizing the expected outcomes. Sharing this information is essential to the success of the project and to future dissemination of its learnings, extension of its scope, and sustainability (Gido & Clements, 2015).

Evaluation involves reviewing overall project outcomes, performance of the project team, and stakeholder involvement. Did the project deliver the benefits, meet the objectives, produce the deliverables on time and within budget, and use resources wisely? Did the action plan follow the expected pathway (management processes)? Was the project team able to determine key project achievements, failures, and lessons learned to inform future direction? Referring back to the initiation and planning phases, the project team considers how the project performed relative to the description in the business case, objectives (outcomes), quality targets, timelines, budget, and resources. Did the internal and external (research) evidence used to support the interventions (action) work as anticipated? How does this contribute to the larger system? What are the implications for spread and dissemination? Within the overall summary (executive summary), key elements to include are the major achievements (positive effects/benefits), failures (what did not go as planned), and lessons learned and recommendations (next steps). A successful project management plan and model can inform future projects, serving as a guide (template) for ongoing deliberate work of the project team (Gido & Clements, 2015).

▶ Planning for Implementation

A successful implementation begins with the creation of an executable work plan. The implementation project manager is responsible for crafting the details of this plan—an activity that includes defining goals, objectives, and strategies; developing a timeline; establishing project milestones; and matching project tasks with resources. During the planning process, it is also important to consider overall aims, goals, outcomes, costs, and budgets simultaneously.

▶ Developing a Project Charter

Developing a written charter is one method of providing clarity regarding the goals, objectives, and timelines for a project plan. In addition, a charter is a key aspect of improvement in that it establishes the written plan for an improvement intervention and defines the small test-of-change methods that will be used. In health care and specific to improvement teams, the elements of the charter provide the framework or scaffold for the project plan and the improvement team that will be responsible for initiating the plan (Richter & Scudder, 2014).

To create a functional written charter, the first step is to form an interprofessional team whose members will work together cohesively to meet the improvement plan or project goals. A team is formed based on the needs of the project to be completed. The skills of the members selected are those necessary to provide insight into the most efficient and effective methods to meet the project goals.

The team's initial composition may be expanded over time as the project goals and objectives are fleshed out and if additional representation is deemed necessary. However, it is essential that those persons involved in the work be the individuals most directly affected by the work to be accomplished as well as those who have the authority and responsibility to effect change.

Once a team is formed, the members of the group operationally define all aspects of the project plan and establish the written charter. A written charter may be developed using an established template that provides a "checklist" of all essential elements for developing, implementing, and evaluating an intervention or improvement project (Richter & Scudder, 2014). Key elements of a written charter may include items such as a project title that clearly articulates the context of the project, dates of project initiation and completion, a listing of team members who will participate in the project, and executive sponsors and team leaders to address the "demographics" of the project. Other sections of the charter may include, but are not limited to, a methodological framework for completing the project; a section providing data and operational definitions for **metrics** used; a section on literature appraisal and synthesis for concepts relevant to the topic and the interventions envisioned; a section for process mapping and any other analyses performed to provide context or direction for the project (e.g., analyses such as policy assessments and strengths, weaknesses, opportunities, and threats [SWOT] assessments); and a defined project plan with numbered "steps," resources needed, timelines (for initiation and completion of steps), assigned accountabilities, interventions, and evaluations for the steps and the overall plan. Additional items that are relevant to the charter may include items such an evaluation and recommendations section as well as a plan for dissemination and sustainability of improvements or interventions.

In summary, the charter should clearly articulate the goals and objectives of the defined improvement effort or project. With a written, clear, well-defined charter, there is less room for ambiguity of goals and interpretation errors of the project plan. Moreover, a clearly defined charter assists in decreasing project scope creep. Therefore, it is recommended that a written charter be clearly defined using some degree of standardization and consistency of elements (Richter & Scudder, 2014).

▶ Model for Improvement

One methodological framework that may be used in project planning and as the underpinnings of the written charter is the Model for Improvement (MFI; Langley et al., 2009). The MFI provides a strong foundation and plan for any improvement effort or intervention. Using the three guiding questions of the MFI may assist the project team in clearly articulating the goals, aims, and/or objectives of the project:

1. What am I trying to accomplish?
2. How will I know a change is an improvement?
3. Which changes can I implement that will result in an improvement?

These three questions provide clarity of purpose and form the central components for a project plan (Langley et al., 2009).

The initial guiding question is central to providing the goal of the project. What is the overall goal or objective that the group should work toward? Sometimes, answering this question is more difficult than one would imagine. Indeed, projects that are broad in scope may have many smaller subprojects that need to be completed before a goal representing a broader perspective may be accomplished. The reverse may also occur. A smaller project may mushroom into one with a broader, more global view of or perspective on a process. For example, a team may form to understand the transfer of a patient with a pain pump through a hospital, but upon better understanding of the elements of the project, the goal may change to become standardizing "pain management processes" throughout a facility. Clearly defining the ultimate goal is central to developing a project plan that will meet that goal.

The second question of the MFI provides the evaluation criteria for the improvement efforts or intervention that is being implemented and tested. It is necessary to provide an analytical assessment of an improvement effort to demonstrate measurable results. Defined measurable criteria are articulated by operationally defining the metrics that will be used to achieve baseline measurements and postintervention or postimplementation measurements. Operational definitions are necessary to clearly define a numerical measure, as well as the tools or methods used to perform that measurement. For example, when defining a rate for "patient falls," it is necessary to define the term "fall" as well as the means by which the rate will be measured. What are the numerator and the denominator for the rate, and are there specific inclusion and exclusion criteria that should be used? Evaluation of an improvement will guide the process of either disseminating the intervention established or changing the plan and revising the implementation if the goals and objectives set for the improvement are not met (Langley et al., 2009).

The final question in the MFI seeks to define the intervention that will be used to improve the process being evaluated. In this step, the team envisions a change that will lead to an improvement in the outcome defined by the measure or evaluation in the second guiding question. For example, if the team intended to improve the patient fall rate, then an intervention specific to falls would be developed. This may include processes such as developing and implementing a more accurate, evidence-based "falls risk assessment" tool on a nursing unit. The intervention is first defined and operationalized and then implemented and evaluated (Langley et al., 2009).

The three guiding questions of the MFI "set the stage" or provide the foundation for "testing" change that may lead to improving a process. Small tests of change are often accomplished through the use of a plan–do–study–act (PDSA) cycle. The PDSA cycle is the engine for change that one would use to *plan* an improvement effort, *do* or implement the plan, *study* the results of the implemented plan, and *act* upon the results by either disseminating the project or changing the plan and repeating in an iterative fashion. Small test-of-change, PDSA cycles are a method for testing improvement interventions in a systematic and focused manner.

Use of the MFI and PDSA approach may provide standardization of improvement efforts within a project plan and should be included in the written charter. The articulation and definition of these elements provide clarity for project efforts and may assist in focusing a project or improvement team on the project goals and objectives (Langley et al., 2009).

The project manager leads the team in conducting a SWOT analysis, in which the team identifies strengths and weaknesses (internal forces) as well as opportunities and threats (external forces). The strengths and opportunities are positive forces that can be exploited to efficiently implement a project. Weaknesses and threats may hamper project implementation if they are not considered in light of the overall aims and context of the project. Many organizations simultaneously conduct a needs assessment and a SWOT analysis and then compare findings. The needs assessment focuses on a summary of the following areas:

- Descriptions of the qualitative and quantitative data that support the need for the project
- The costs, resources, stakeholder buy-in, and work requirements necessary for a successful and meaningful project outcome prior to implementation
- Determination of whether needs are strategically aligned with the organization's mission and overall goals

The information gleaned from the needs assessment is pivotal and requires comprehensive consideration prior to planning and implementing a project. In this step, the role of the implementation project manager transitions into that of risk anticipator, assisting project stakeholders in devising a strategy means of overcoming potential barriers. It is best to begin with the end in mind. That is, what is the expectation for quality outcomes when undertaking a project initiative? Lighter (2011), for example, identified the need for stakeholders to consider the value proposition when implementing a project. More specifically, he proposed the following formula to calculate value:

Value = quality/cost

According to Skor (2013), establishing a substantive value proposition is critical to successful companies and projects undertaken to meet operational goals. This step starts the journey from the inception of an idea to completion of the project. Skor defines a value proposition as a positioning statement that outlines the benefits provided for the agent or company and explains how those benefits uniquely address the need. The target market, the problem to be solved, and why this solution is better than the alternatives are other information included in a well-stated value proposition. The creation of a compelling value proposition includes four steps: (1) defining, (2) evaluating, (3) measuring, and (4) building.

In the *defining* step, the team provides the information that determines if the problem is worth solving. Skor (2013) describes the four U's as being significant to defining the value proposition. If the answers are "yes" to the majority of these questions, it is likely that the project planners are moving in the right direction toward a compelling value proposition:

1.   *Is the concern Unworkable?* If there were inaction in regard to a real problem, perhaps someone gets fired without addressing the issue, or you lose a major customer, this would likely direct the need to finding a solution. For example, the person who may be fired would likely be an excellent internal champion of the project.
2.   *Is fixing the problem Unavoidable?* If regulatory or accreditation issues are on the table, that factor drives fundamental requirements for compliance and accountability issues. Answering "yes" to this question would likely identify the group that should serve as a champion for the project.
3.   *Is the concern Urgent?* Is this concern a top priority to the system? Without attention to the issue, would you likely lose market share or other major resources? If the answer is "yes," the corporate suite's attention will likely be drawn to the concern.
4.   *Is the problem Underserved?* If there appears to be no (or limited) solution to the problem you want to address, you may be identifying a segment of the market (or white space) that would increase your organization's value. If you answer "yes" to this question, then your company may be primed to increase its market share.

Another tool that Skor (2013) recommends is qualifying the problem as "BLAC and White." BLAC is an acronym standing for Blatant, Latent, Aspirational, and Critical; White refers to the "white space" that the projects capitalize on as an opportunity for growth. Skor notes that concerns or problems that are blatant and critical are more likely to attract attention because they tend to stand in the way of doing business and are more acute than latent or aspirational problems. When a problem is latent, it is generally unacknowledged; aspirational problems are considered optional and are often the most difficult to consider in a fast-paced, frenetic market.

The second step, *evaluating*, seeks to determine whether the solution is unique or compelling enough to continue the effort in the planning. Once the problem is defined as critical for pursuing, the team must identify what is unique and compelling about a solution to this problem. Skor (2013) offers a useful approach in the context of the three D's. The three D's provide a thoughtful approach to considering the unique combination of Discontinuous innovation, Defensible technology, and a Disruptive business model that makes a solution compelling to the team and its target—a possibly skeptical market. A *discontinuous* innovation provides transformative benefits over the status quo by viewing the problem through different lenses. *Defensible* technology encompasses intellectual property that can be protected to develop a barrier to entry and an unfair competitive advantage. *Disruptive* business models can catalyze the growth of the venture by enabling its employees to understand the value and cost rewards. While "faster, cheaper, and better" may also be a useful metric, evaluating the three D's can expand thinking about a potential breakthrough.

Skor's (2013) third step, *measure,* considers the gain/pain ratio of potential adoption of a solution to a problem. This ratio compares the gain that solution will deliver to the target market versus the pain and cost required for the solution's adoption. Skor reports that he looks for nondisruptive innovations—that is, those technologies that offer game-changing benefits yet require only minimal modifications to current processes and systems. Nondisruptive introduction is essential to new projects because the gains they deliver will be discounted by the risks associated with altering the current system. A successful venture delivers an order-of-magnitude improvement over the status quo. According to Skor, if you are not able to deliver a 10-fold gain/pain promise, stakeholders and the target market will typically default to "do nothing" rather than bearing the risk of working with you. To overcome this reluctance to change, you will need to assure that your innovation is measurable to a degree that change is notable.

Skor's (2013) final step, *build,* involves moving from defining, evaluating, and measuring to actually creating the value proposition. Skor recommends the following framework for the *building* step:

1. Who are your stakeholders? Your target customers?
2. Who and what are dissatisfied with your current performance?
3. What will this new strategy (product) be?
4. What will be provided? What provides key problem-solving capability?
5. What is unlike your product? What is the product (intervention) alternative?

According to Skor (2013), the most important consideration is the individual (*you*) that creates the value proposition and carries out the strategies. You, the project planner, are core to *your* value proposition. How do *you* understand and deliver uniquely? Which kind of disruptive business model can *you* bring? Skor describes being true to *yourself* as a thought leader as a means to ensure that *you* will go far.

Inherent in the planning process is the development of an implementation strategy. The implementation strategy is meant to focus on the process from a stakeholder perspective and should be approved prior to execution. The most common implementation strategy is the phased approach for a project (Glaser, 2009). This approach is relatively safe for the organization because it allows the project team members to reassess their progress after each project phase is operationalized. For example, in a project to reduce catheter-acquired urinary tract infections (CAUTIs), phases may include determination of the extent of the problem, use of data to drive the urgency to act (magnitude of problem), outcomes to be measured, implementation strategies, and evaluation protocols.

A key document in the implementation phase is the project charter. The project charter is an agreement between the organization providing the service and the stakeholder requesting the service and receiving the deliverables (Lewis, 2005). It includes a comprehensive description of the project, a list of anticipated project team members, and those members' specific roles and responsibilities in the project. Also included in the charter is the level of authority for the project manager and the project outcomes. The project charter outlines the scope and measures of success and includes formal signatures for project authorization and approval. This process is critical to building consensus on project goals and documents communication between project stakeholders.

For example, a project aimed at reducing CAUTIs on an acute surgical unit might involve the clinical nurse leader (CNL), the infection control nurse, a patient representative, and staff nurses. The CNL may take the lead as project manager, outlining particular roles of each member (e.g., observing how patients' urinary catheters are handled during transport, monitoring the number of catheters inserted and discontinued). Tasks related to setting up communication channels, meeting times, and review tools may also be established and delegated by the CNL. While other team members are intimately involved in the implementation of the project and have an active voice in all project-related measures, the CNL is the project manager, but they cannot and should not be expected to produce the project outcomes alone.

Another phase of the project implementation may revolve around the action plan (based on the best available evidence) that delineates particular strategies. The action plan includes the following elements:

- How evidence-based interventions will be used to improve the system (system change) and practice.
- The *how* to accomplish the stated purpose.
- The collaboration and teamwork required to implement the project, its sustainability, and its relevance to an existing program or mission.
- Information flow processes (informatics and technology).
- Interventions that will focus on educating others about the project and means by which the information provided will guide stakeholders throughout the implementation phase and result in the stated project goal/aim.
- Descriptions of the theoretical or conceptual underpinnings and their relevance to the overall project and program mission.
- How organizational and cultural dynamics will be addressed.
- Anticipated impacts that the project will have and explanation of how findings will close gaps identified by the SWOT analysis and needs assessment.
- Time-specific milestones.

An evaluation phase to measure the success of actions taken is important to determine the efficacy of the plan. An evaluation plan includes the following elements:

- Methods and metrics for evaluating the project.
- Timelines and data milestones.
- Measurement types that include structure, process, and outcome.
- Metrics that gather evidence relevant to stakeholders and the system, are scientifically sound, and are associated with processes that can be modified through reasonable methods and procedures.
- Lessons learned, barriers that were overcome during the implementation phase, and strategies used to overcome the barriers that could further inform the project.

▶ Micro-, Meso-, and Macro-Collaboration

Collaboration across organizational stakeholders requires communication, commitment, accountability, and continuity (McElmurry et al., 2009). To ensure that a new initiative is realized to its full potential, stakeholders must see the strategic alignment. Administrative support for a project may enhance successful implementation and sustainability. For example, a project for reducing CAUTIs aimed at reducing patients' discomfort and costs of care serves to advance the mission of the organization. In particular, it addresses the overall mission of quality—that is, safe care. The implementation project manager translates to stakeholders how existing business processes would be improved with project implementation. Project stakeholders (project sponsors, decision makers, and leaders) in a healthcare organization publicly endorsing the project may underscore the importance of the project's purpose.

In terms of the implementation of a project, collaboration with stakeholders is priceless. It is important to involve organizational stakeholders from the beginning, perform intermittent progress checks, be responsive to concerns, and address risks throughout implementation. At the point of implementation, the project manager ensures resource needs are clear and project risks are reviewed and validated. Stakeholder expectations must be managed during implementation through continued focus on the strategic goals of the project (McElmurry et al., 2009). Structure, process, and outcome indicators are continually evaluated to assure that resources are being used efficiently and effectively. Meetings to share progress and lessons learned—for example, actual reductions in CAUTI rates—will further enhance the credibility of the project team's work.

▶ Communicate, Communicate, and Communicate

In addition to planning and collaboration, the other fundamental element of implementation is communication. The purpose of communications management is to share the right information, at the right time, with the right people, and in the right format. Good communications management requires expending effort on sharing information, which contributes to project success; conversely, lack of information can lead to failure. Most importantly, the project manager must identify the correct target audience for different categories of communications.

Strong communication must be accompanied by mutual trust. Both formal and informal methods can be used to disseminate information. Formal communication methods follow well-defined, systematic procedures, whereas informal communications are casual and more extemporaneous. Weekly status reports containing information about progress and issues are examples of a formal communication tool. Examples of informal communication include voice mail, email, and text messages. An effective and perhaps an efficient method of conveying information within a team is face-to-face conversation.

The implementation plan should be circulated to all stakeholders involved in the project. The implementation project manager must communicate continually to reinforce the messages related to that plan and make sure everyone is ready when implementation begins.

The management of communication is implemented through three essential processes:

- *Identification:* The process of identifying information to be shared, when it should be distributed, who should receive it, and how it should be prepared.
- *Reporting:* The process of collecting and preparing the information.
- *Distribution:* The process of disseminating the information and, for formal communications, storing the information in the project archive.

▶ Change Management

Change management is possibly the most important factor in the implementation process. For example, when a healthcare organization is adopting a new clinical or financial information system, its business processes will undergo significant changes, so there will be a definite learning curve. The change process must be actively managed. Change management may be led by someone external to the organization, possibly a consultant, and begins at the same time as implementation. The individual or group of individuals charged with handling this task should collaborate with the implementation project manager and project stakeholders to craft a change management blueprint tailored for the organization.

An effective change management technique is for one department to test the new approach before it is rolled out more broadly. In other words, rather than a big-bang start, it is often more productive to begin with one unit or department trying out the project initiative. A staged approach allows the implementation project manager and stakeholders to monitor the initiative at work on a small scale and react to any resulting issues. This steady progression generates confidence and understanding throughout the organization, building buy-in for the project. This gradual process of integration can be replicated with employees as well. They are encouraged to start off slowly and build their knowledge and confidence related to the project initiative.

Faculty members from the University of South Alabama College of Nursing developed a model that visually illustrates the intersecting aspects of a system change project that can assist organizations and students when planning and implementing a project (**FIGURE 10-1**). Questions are posed for each intersecting aspect that can guide the implementation of the system change project. The intersecting aspects and accompanying questions are presented here:

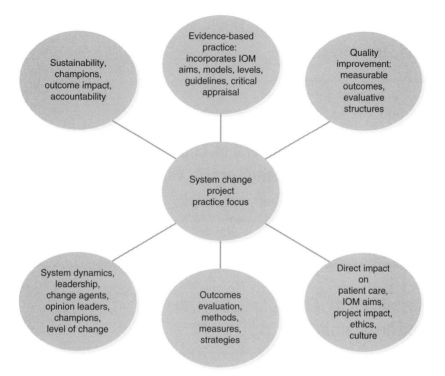

FIGURE 10-1 System Change Project Intersecting Aspects

Evidence-Based Practice: Incorporates IOM Aims, Models, Levels, Guidelines, and Critical Appraisal

- Is there a model or framework of how evidence is managed?
- Are level(s) identified?
- Is there a critical appraisal mechanism?

Quality Improvement: Measurable Outcomes and Evaluative Structures

- Is a model/framework plan in place?
- What is the quality improvement process?

Direct Impact on Patient Care, IOM Aims, Project Impact, Ethics, and Culture

- Are the aims clearly defined?
- What is the direct impact on patient care?

Outcomes Evaluation, Methods, Measures, and Strategies

- Are outcomes defined?
- Are measures to be evaluated identified?
- Are methods to evaluate outcomes defined?

System Dynamics, Leadership, Change Agents, Opinion Leaders, Champions, and Level of Change

- Is there a conceptual/theoretical framework identified?
- Is it integrated into the project plan?
- Which system(s) are to be changed?
- Who are the change agents? Opinion leaders? Change champions?
- Is this an incremental change? Transformational change? How do you know?

Sustainability, Champions, Outcome Impact, and Accountability

- Do long-term plans exist?
- Which plans are in place to maintain sustainability?

▶ Resistance to Change Is a Reality—Embrace It

Training and education play an important role in overcoming resistance in the adoption of new organizational initiatives. Research has revealed that adult learners have the capability to grasp new information early in the implementation phase of a project (Bond, 2006). The implementation project manager must collaborate with educational resources within the organization to develop training materials in the planning process of this project. Equally important is the support of decision makers and leadership in providing these resources to support project efforts.

▶ Post-Project Monitoring and Evaluation

Projects should be continuously evaluated for quality and appropriateness. Adjustments can then be made at the time of discovery, instead of waiting until the end of project implementation (Kitzmiller, Hunt, & Sproat, 2006). With such an approach, the project may have more minor, smaller adjustments instead of larger, costlier swings in project scope and direction.

Postimplementation reviews can be conducted to identify value achievement progress and the steps still needed to achieve maximum gain. It is extremely rare for healthcare organizations to revisit their investments to determine whether promised value was actually achieved (Glaser, 2009). Some organizations believe that once the implementation is over and the change settles in, value will automatically be achieved

(Glaser, 2009). In reality, it is wise for healthcare organizations to conduct reviews of projects periodically to evaluate progress.

Postimplementation reviews support the achievement of value by signaling leadership interest in ensuring the delivery of results, identifying the steps to ensure value, and reinforcing accountability for results. The reviews also answer questions such as the following:

- Which goals were expected to be met at the time the project was approved?
- How close has the organization come to achieving those project goals?
- How much has the organization invested in the project, and how does it compare with the original budget?
- If the organization had to implement the project again, what would it do differently?

Monitoring is an important component of the implementation phase to ensure that the project is implemented per the schedule. It is a continuous process that should be put in place before project implementation starts. Monitoring activities should be executed by all individuals and institutions that have an interest (stakeholders) in the project. To efficiently implement a project, the people planning and implementing it should plan for all the interrelated stages from the beginning. Metrics are also important to ensure that activities are implemented as planned. They help the implementation project manager measure how well project milestones and goals are being achieved. As such, the monitoring activities should appear on the work plan and should involve all stakeholders. If project activities are not going well, arrangements should be made to identify the problems as early as possible so that they can be corrected.

Organizations should benchmark their performance in achieving value against the performance of like organizations (Glaser, 2009). These benchmarks may focus on process performance, using data to inform activities ranging from resource allocation to instructional practice. Stakeholders, especially project sponsors, should understand the accountability they have for the successful completion of the project. There should be an agreed-upon set of metrics that will be used to track value delivery. These metrics should complement the metrics used to evaluate project implementation.

▶ Project Implementation Challenges and Risks

Project implementation can be improved by asking a series of questions, including seeking to know the activities that produce expected project outputs, inquiring about the sequencing and time frames for the planned activities, and determining who will be responsible for carrying out each activity. A number of tools can be used to monitor these activities such as a Gantt chart, Critical Path Method (CPM) or Network analysis, and Project Evaluation and Review Techniques (PERT). For example, the Gantt chart is also referred to as the progress chart showing the timing of project activities using horizontal bars. The Gantt chart is one of the techniques of project scheduling that illustrates the frequency of activities and outlines the period of time for implementation. Using a Gantt chart can assist with determining the parts or implementation phases of the project, the sequencing of associated activities to be carried out, the estimated time required for each activity, and listing activities carried out at the same time and identifying those to be carried out sequentially. Constructing a Gantt chart involves a horizontal axis (time) and a vertical axis (activities). Specifically, bars are entered to determine the time period designated for each activity and progression at any particular point in time (Bañuls, López, Turoff, & Tejedor, 2017).

Tools for implementation can facilitate successful projects. Other considerations for successful projects include political commitment, simplicity of design, careful preparation, good management, and involvement of beneficiaries/community. Conversely, factors and problems that lead to failure of projects may be financial problems, management problems, technical problems, and political problems. Other factors include poor scheduling of projects leading to delays in implementation, misallocation of funds, delay and sometimes lack of counterpart funding, lack of accountability and transparency, bureaucracy in decision-making, and selfishness/nepotism/favoritism by some project managers. Additional implementation problems may be weak monitoring systems, policy changes, migration of beneficiaries, lack of teamwork, and lack of incentives for implementers (Thompson & Cox, 2017).

Many potential challenges and risks may arise in the development, planning, and implementation of projects. Some of the common ones include funding and the management of stakeholders. If numerous stakeholders will be directly involved in the project, at least some political challenges will undoubtedly be encountered. Another frequent implementation challenge is the lack of communication among stakeholders, leadership, and the implementation project manager. Such miscommunication creates divergence in perceptions of critical initiatives that have great potential to benefit a healthcare organization, which in turn could lead to quality and safety risks.

Some common reasons for project implementation failure are poor communication with leadership and stakeholders, organizational resistance to change, scope creep, lack of project ownership and champion, and shifts in organizational priorities. The recommended approach for achieving implementation success is the incorporation of **agility** into the project process (Kitzmiller et al., 2006). Agility is a concept that encourages flexibility, adaptation, and continuous learning as a part of the implementation process. The agility process accepts the complexity of a problem and addresses it through frequent inspection, responding with a flexible approach of constant adaption (Kitzmiller et al., 2006). Agility considers the complexity of the problems faced in the current healthcare environment and enhances traditional implementation techniques.

▶ Summary

- Implementation is the final process of moving the solution from development to production status.
- Successful implementation begins with an executable plan.
- SWOT analysis and needs assessment are critical to successful project implementation.
- Project charters identify outcomes that can be tracked.
- Collaboration requires communication among and between all stakeholders.
- A system change project considers several aspects that impact practice outcomes.

Reflection Questions

1. What are two aspects of project planning that will ensure success? Compare them to situations in daily practice.
2. Which factors should be considered when dealing with external forces and barriers that can impede project implementation?

3. Consider a project that you have implemented. Which strengths, weakness, threats, and opportunities did you identify when implementing the project?

References

Bañuls, V. A., López, C., Turoff, M., & Tejedor, F. (2017). Predicting the impact of multiple risks on project performance: A scenario-based approach. *Project Management Journal, 48*(5), 95–114.

Bond, G. E. (2006). Lessons learned from the implementation of web-based nursing intervention. *Computers in Nursing, 24*(2), 66–74.

Gido, J., & Clements, J. P. (2015). *Successful project management* (6th ed.). Boston, MA: Cengage Learning.

Glaser, J. (2009). A strategy for ensuring a project delivers value. *Healthcare Financial Management, 63*(7), 28–31.

Institute for Healthcare Improvement (IHI). (2017). *IHI Improvement Capability Self-Assessment Tool.* Retrieved from http://www.ihi.org/resources/Pages/Tools/IHIImprovementCapabilitySelfAssessmentTool.aspx

Kitzmiller, R., Hunt, E., & Sproat, S. (2006). Adopting best practices: Agility moves from software development to healthcare project management. *Computers in Nursing, 24*(2), 75–82.

Krigsman, M. (2011, March 15). CIO analysis: Why 37 percent of projects fail. *ZD Net.* Retrieved from http://www.zdnet.com/article/cio-analysis-why-37-percent-of-projects-fail

Langley, G. J., Moen, R. D., Nolan, K. M., Nolan, T. W., Norman, C. L., & Provost, L. P. (2009). *The improvement guide: A practical approach to enhancing organizational performance* (2nd ed.). San Francisco, CA: Jossey-Bass.

Lewis, J. (2005). *Project planning, scheduling, and control.* New York, NY: McGraw-Hill.

Lighter, D. E. (2011). *Advanced performance improvement in health care.* Sudbury, MA: Jones & Bartlett.

McElmurry, B. J., McCreary, L. L., Park, C. G., Ramos, L., Martinez, E., Parikh, R., . . . Fogelfeld, L. (2009). Implementation, outcomes, and lessons learned from a collaborative primary health care program to improve diabetes care among urban Latino populations. *Health Promotion Practice, 10*(2), 293–302.

Phelan, B., & Stockwell, C. (2014). Are your projects delivering business value? *Bright Hub Project Management.* Retrieved from http://www.brighthubpm.com/project-planning/128738-are-your-projects-delivering-business-value

Richter, L., & Scudder, R. (2014). What is a project charter? *Bright Hub Project Management.* Retrieved from http://www.brighthubpm.com/project-planning/5161-what-is-a-project-charter

Roussel, L., & Dearman, C. (2009). *DNP project plan model.* Unpublished work documents in DNP program development.

Skor, M. (2013, June 14). Four steps to building a compelling value proposition. *Forbes.* Retrieved from http://www.forbes.com/sites/michaelskok/2013/06/14/4-steps-to-building-a-compelling-value-proposition

Thompson, S., & Cox, E. (2017). How coaching is used and understood by project managers in organizations. *Project Management Journal, 48*, 64–77.

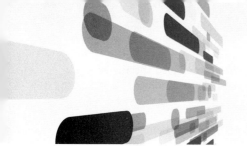

Case Exemplar

▶ Case Study 1

LPN-BSN: An Innovative Articulation Model

K. Michele Lyons

Background

The Patient Protection and Affordable Care Act, aging of the U.S. population, and the nursing faculty shortage will all contribute to the expected nursing shortage in the United States. This shortage, in conjunction with the identified need by the Institute of Medicine (2010) for seamless transfer opportunities to allow nurses to enhance their education, prompted the development of an interagency collaborative project between a community college and a 4-year university. This project will provide students with an alternative method to enter the workforce so as to meet the needs of the nursing shortage as well as provide students with opportunities to further their education.

This interagency collaborative project was modeled after an existing partnership between the community college and the university. Students who require remediation or do not meet the university's admission requirements are admitted into the program. The courses are offered through the community college and are held on the university campus. Once the student has met the program's requirements, the student seamlessly transfers to the university to continue his or her education. The results of this program have demonstrated that students are more likely to successfully transfer when the classes are held on the university's campus and a clearly outlined matriculation plan has been developed.

Objectives

The purpose of this project is to develop and implement an accelerated licensed practical nurse (LPN) program to increase the nursing workforce and provide a seamless transition to a bachelor of science in nursing (BSN) program. The program outcomes are intended to increase the nursing workforce by developing graduates from an accelerated program who are as academically successful as their traditional counterparts and have the same professional attributes as their traditional counterparts.

Methods

The accelerated LPN program began in January 2014 and was expected to produce graduates in December 2014. The students are attending classes on the university campus and being exposed to information about matriculation into BSN opportunities at the university as well as the advantages of gaining a BSN for future career advancement. These students were required to have completed specific general education coursework from a 4-year university prior to being admitted.

Results

Demographic data, including preadmission test scores, are being collected for descriptive purposes. Academic performance will be measured using the following outcomes: National Council Licensure Examination for Practical Nurses (NCLEX-PN) scores, Assessment Technologies Institute Comprehensive Indicator scores, and final grade-point averages. The Nurses Professional Values Scale–Revised (NPVS-R), derived from the American Nurses Association's *Code of Ethics for Nursing*, is being utilized to assess the students' ethical values (American Nurses Association & Fowler, 2008). The expectation is that no difference will be found between the accelerated and traditional LPN students' academic performance and ethical values.

Conclusions

The success of this program will potentially impact nursing education and build a stronger, more diverse workforce. Nursing students should have access to advanced career opportunities within an academic system that allows seamless transfer opportunities.

Reflection Questions

1. How was the need determined to initiate this innovative educational program?
2. Who were the major stakeholders?
3. How was the project conceptualized?
4. How were the program outcomes developed?

References

American Nurses Association, & Fowler, M. D. M. (2008). *Guide to the code of ethics for nurses: Interpretation and application*. Silver Spring, MD: American Nurses Association.

Institute of Medicine. (2010). *The future of nursing: Leading change, advancing health*. Retrieved from http://books.nap.edu/openbook.php?record_id=12956&page=R1

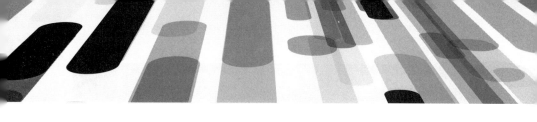

CHAPTER 11

Role of Information Technology in Project Planning and Management

James L. Harris
Todd Harlan

CHAPTER OBJECTIVES

1. Describe the importance of information technology as an enabler when assessing needs and planning evidence-based clinical projects in today's healthcare environment.
2. Identify key stakeholders, partnerships, and their respective roles in developing information technology that supports clinical projects, enterprises, and their management.
3. Examine the significance of key information technology core competencies and skill sets for successful project plans and management in a global society.
4. Explain the value of linking projects to information systems for enhanced functionality, data conversion, and data utility.
5. Examine the role of data integrity, security, protection of human subjects, and regulatory agencies within the context of planning projects and their management.

KEY TERMS

Big data
Clinical enterprise
Data integrity
Human-subject protection
Information management
Information technology

Privacy
Security
Small data
Stakeholder
Value

ROLES

Educator
Leader

Partner
Team member

PROFESSIONAL VALUES

Efficiency
Integrity
Performance

Privacy
Quality

CORE COMPETENCIES

Communication
Design

Information technology knowledge
Management

▶ Introduction

The advent of the Patient Protection and Affordable Care Act, also known more simply as the Affordable Care Act (ACA), represents the largest change to the U.S. healthcare system since the genesis of the Medicare and Medicaid programs in 1965 (Institute of Medicine [IOM], 2001, 2011). The U.S. healthcare system has experienced and will continue to undergo numerous changes as more Americans seek care. How the healthcare industry responds to changes in technology, impending care mandates, reimbursement models, and the information age will be driven by knowledgeable consumers and leaders who are able to make informed decisions. The momentum needed for survival will be shaped by how well and how accurately needs are assessed, systems leverage technology to improve outcomes, and evidence-based projects are initiated. Quantum leaps in efficiency and effectiveness will be realized as the diffusion of technology drives projects and determines the role that the information specialist will play in the process (Geibert, 2017). However, such projects will only be as effective as the partnership that is built with a transformative clinical project manager.

The clinical project manager must be poised to support the project activities with necessary tools, issue management, and coordination (Gallagher, 2012). Ownership of any clinical project is given to clinical **stakeholders** by reinforcing that it is not an **information technology** or support project but rather a clinically driven project with interprofessional participation as a cornerstone (J. P. Lewis, 2011). Ongoing human activities are needed for data conversion and the spread of knowledge. Otherwise, as projects mature, the identified project aims and outcomes will not be realized. The merits of information technology will also be limited in such unsuccessful projects, and improvements in **value** obtained by consumers, payers, and accreditation agencies will be less than optimal (Lighter, 2011).

▶ Information Technology as an Enabler for Clinical Project Success

The availability of electronic networks 24/7 provides access across points of care. Equally, evidence-based data are readily available as clinical projects are envisioned and initiated. But what enables a clinical project's success and its management? While there is no one formula that is guaranteed to ensure the project meets its aims, the use of informatics is a valuable tool in today's evolving technological healthcare environment. Investing in new ways to seize opportunities to mix technology with project ideas is important as nurses and other providers interact with clinical informatics departments. The potential for all staff to enhance practice, solve clinical problems, and improve care has paved the way for informatics. Interprofessional care teams of the 21st century will be ineffective without a solid base of informatics, computers, and information technology (Kelly, 2012). Likewise, all individuals engaged in clinical project development will experience a similar void if this knowledge base is lacking. Understanding the scope of informatics and technology provides context. It serves as an enabler when identifying needs that structure project aims, guides related processes, and ultimately shapes the outcomes (National Advisory Council on Nurse Education and Practice, 1997). Leveraging the skills of informatics specialists when developing new projects and adopting measurement tools can optimize iterative processes that limit workarounds. The creation of a digital culture for healthcare organizations can be achieved (Morrison, 2011). Informatics and technological advances provide clinical applications that can process transactions with tools for productivity, business strategies, collaboration, and innovations by exploiting unique technological advances (Shane, 2014).

Now we can answer the earlier question: What enables a project's success and its ongoing management? Numerous individuals and organizations have identified multiple enablers that support many projects, programs, and organizational efficacy and are used daily to improve care (California HealthCare Foundation and First Consulting Group, 2002; DeLaune & Ladner, 2009; Fox, 2011; Stevens & Staley, 2006):

- Computerized order entry
- Electronic health records
- Peer-to-peer health care
- Mobile communication devices
- Securing messaging and email
- Automated documentation templates and clinical reminders
- Medication administration and management systems
- Evidence-based knowledge and information retrieval systems with remote library, smartphone, and Internet resources

- Quality improvement data collection and data summary systems
- Data mining techniques for sorting large data batches
- Webpages for personalizing information
- Disease surveillance systems
- Computerized data encounter archives

These enablers and their supporting information technology (IT) systems have created multiple opportunities that assist providers daily in responding to patient needs. They serve as milestones whereby IT's ability to facilitate past and future project success and ongoing project management can be measured. Freeing staff from repetitive tasks via IT provides more opportunities for staff to engage with patients and engenders a culture of patient-centeredness.

To maximize each of these enablers and IT systems when planning a project, many considerations and data points must be taken into account. The benefits can range from the needs assessment phase to completion of the project and dissemination of results. Big and small data are valuable data sets and are analyzed and integrated into a project design (Beal, 2014). **Big data** is generated from multiple sources and provides a snapshot of what is happening without answering why. It is used to describe, interpret, and predict (Henly, 2014). **Small data** provides information to answer a specific question or address an identified problem. Small data feeds big data by creating new knowledge and care advances (McCartney, 2015).

Two especially important considerations, the organizational mission statement and critical success factors, cannot be dismissed as enablers for project planning. As the project is planned, reviewing the organizational mission statement and linking the project focus to the mission can both directly and indirectly prove beneficial in securing buy-in and support. Examples of the benefits from such links may include financial benefits, meeting quality service and patient and/or employee satisfaction objectives, and continuous opportunities for learning and growth.

Critical success factors (CSF) are those elements that must work effectively to ensure high performance within an organization. For example, CSFs are used to prioritize operational initiatives and assist leaders in choosing the most pressing and relevant activities and projects to initiate and support. Again, being cognizant of these factors and linking them to the project and processes will yield positive outcomes.

▶ Stakeholder and Partner Roles in Information Technology

Identifying and engaging stakeholders continuously during a clinical project is pivotal to that project's success. Similarly, information technology must be an integral part of data retrieval and meaningful use to an organization. As stakeholders participate in a project, whether by engaging in the approval process or by offering encouragement, keeping in mind the need to represent their interests is important to the ongoing phases of any project or **clinical enterprise**. When stakeholders participate, partnerships emerge, ownership is reinforced, and support for the project takes center stage.

An imperative for participation by stakeholders and ongoing partnerships is the commitment and value that information technology development provides and IT's role throughout the project and the organization. The demand for value with any project endeavor will continuously be emphasized, as will the need to invest in value-based

IT if gaps in clinical care are to be filled. End users will assist in communicating the value to stakeholders and the utility of supporting all projects, their implementation, and their sustainability in the long term.

As a student or expert project developer considers and plans new projects or redesigns those that may have previously failed, IT investment and partnerships between project managers and IT departments will create a competitive edge for the organization. However, the magnitude of this effect will depend on how well IT systems are designed and their relationships to other business and organizational metrics. As knowledge is generated and spread, and the information generated in terms of local project outcomes is interconnected with national information resources, variability among data will be minimized. Information exchanges will therefore guide clinical and organizational decisions (Sicotte & Paré, 2010). Opportunities for avoiding and managing risk will be created and deleterious errors reduced. The content of information exchanges will be further strengthened as informatics core competencies and skill sets are developed and utilized and as IT specialists are engaged during all phases of a project.

▶ Informatics Core Competencies and Skill Sets

In today's global environment and economy, IT has become a thread woven throughout all types of organizations. Whether an individual is directly or indirectly involved in patient care or beginning a clinical project, he or she must be armed with a general knowledge of informatics. The need for organizational and care efficiency, for example, requires healthcare team members to review and mine data so that they can design or redesign care delivery models and productivity. Such activities require competency and skills in informatics, both general and advanced. For those individuals with limited informatics knowledge, knowing where to seek assistance is essential if goals are to be attained. This need resonates with one of the IOM's healthcare professional core competencies (utilize informatics); indeed, its fifth healthcare profession core competency is delineated as the ability to "communicate, manage knowledge, mitigate error, and support decision-making using information technology" (IOM, 2003, p. 4). Likewise, the IOM's report *The Future of Nursing* (2011) and the position statement from the Healthcare Information and Management Systems Society (2011) echo the need for nurses to possess informatics competency and skills.

Recognition of the significance of IT core competencies and skills for successful projects and management dates to early work at the University of Maryland that identified three levels of competencies (technical, professional, and advanced) for its multidisciplinary student body (Ball & Douglas, 1989). Grobe's (1988, 1989) seminal work describing informatics competencies for medical students was later modified to create seven levels of informatics competencies for nursing students, also applicable to other allied health disciplines. **BOX 11-1** identifies these seven levels of competencies.

The method used by Grobe made it difficult to confirm that nurses had updated their competencies in this area. Nevertheless, Grobe's work represented a beginning step toward identifying a comprehensive taxonomy of competencies that exist on a continuum ranging from user to modifier to innovator. A further step followed in which a competency grid for each practice domain linked the role functions for each domain (clinical practice, nurse manager, nurse educator, and nurse researcher) with

BOX 11-1 Grobe's Nursing Informatics Competencies for Basic and Graduate Nursing Education

1. Use basic information-handling tools
2. Independently learn about computers and **information management**
3. Use computer systems and access databases
4. Knowledgeably use systems and specialized databases
5. Perceive new applications
6. Build systems for personal applications
7. Tool building

a corresponding range of nursing informatics competencies (technical, professional, and advanced).

For decades, healthcare professionals have advanced their care delivery as new competencies have emerged, including those related to informatics. Likewise, multiple vocabularies have been used to classify care. Given that nurses document care on a 24/7 basis, however, there is no single system used in electronic medical records to record nursing care (Cipriano, 2014). Clark and Lang (1992) identified the key shortcoming associated with this practice: "If we cannot name it, we cannot control it, finance it, teach it, research it, or put [it] into public policy" (p. 109). While advancing clinical competencies is necessary to meet care demands, the ongoing development of informatics competencies will be required for successful data management. Educators must provide guided opportunities for students and graduates to develop meaningful projects that are data-driven and evidence-based. This need is clearly apparent when one reviews baccalaureate, master's, and doctor of nursing practice end-of-program competencies (American Association of Colleges of Nursing [AACN], 2006, 2008, 2011).

The challenges of the digital age call for others to perceive roles differently and to express those perspectives in ways that best fit a sociotechnical culture (Porter-O'Grady & Malloch, 2015). This endeavor encourages transformational thinking and action spanning all disciplines and cultures. Meaningful projects that add value and guide quality and the delivery of safe care will be possible with informed users and managers of data as projects are formed, implemented, replicated, and linked to information systems.

▶ The Value of Linking Projects to Information Systems

From the inception to dissemination of any project, its value must be considered. Value must be attainable and measured to ensure that the resources allotted to a project did, in fact, advance the mission and vision of the organization. Likewise, the value to stakeholders must be measurable and attainable, as they are the end recipients of a clinical project.

Measuring value can be complex and requires the use of data from various sources. The data must be informative, relevant, and sensitive to the intent of a project so that a difference is evident in desired outcomes. Meeting this standard requires one to link the project to information systems; otherwise, changing inefficient processes will be more difficult, and the value produced may be questionable (Nelson, Batalden, & Godfrey, 2007). Remembering that all healthcare systems are embedded in complex systems, and that all things intersect and are in constant interactions with one another, is important for the success of any project endeavor. Complexity science supports this notion and can inform how value is determined and documented. Linking projects to the correct metrics and information system will aid in measuring the project's value (Porter-O'Grady & Malloch, 2015).

Information systems are the "nervous system" for meaningful projects and can provide the context for how a project benefits practice, education, quality improvement, management, and policy. When planning the project, one must select those metrics that will measure specific outcomes based on the project's aim. Aligning the metrics to the correct information system will isolate the effect of the project based on desired outcomes and allows for greater functionality, conversion, and utility of the data gathered. Conversely, failure to ensure such alignment is a common flaw in the design process. Metrics that effectively measure success extend beyond business and strategic goals and are linked to stakeholders who have a vested interest in the success of any project. Those metrics must be specific and quantifiable (A. Lewis, 2011). To further illustrate this point, consider the example of a clinical success metric identified in **TABLE 11-1**.

For health informatics projects, Gallagher (2012) identified five phases that provide valuable information for personnel ranging from the novice to the expert. First, the initiation phase should involve an informaticist when developing project requirements, scope, and vendor contracts and requirements. This can eliminate incongruity between customer expectations and the product. Second, the planning phase includes the determination of tasks to ensure design, workflow, and barrier identification. Third, execution begins, and the end users of the project are involved as products are tested, adjustments are made, super users are identified, and education is continuous. The fourth stage involves monitoring to ensure all deliverables are met and issues are resolved. Otherwise, the progress of the project can be jeopardized, including the budget. In the final phase, closing, all open issues are resolved and any additional modifications completed for a smooth and effective project that will have meaningful use to all involved.

TABLE 11-1 Clinical Success Metric	
Success Metric	**Attainable, Measurable Outcomes from Information System**
Improved quality, safe, and efficient patient care processes	■ Medication order entry errors (pharmacy, medical, and nursing services) ■ Timely signing and verification of emergency verbal orders (medical and nursing services, health information management, pharmacy, and quality improvement)

Healthcare-related projects require the involvement of a variety of individuals; moreover, to ensure that a project is meaningful, the best available tools must be selected. If quality, safety, efficiency, and continuous improvement are to be achieved with the initiation of any project and its subsequent sustainment, ongoing measurement is pivotal to success. Donabedian (1978) provided an excellent way to characterize medical quality, based on structure, process, and outcome measures. Using Donabedian's model, quality improvement teams consistently use these measures to guide the development of metrics that are linked to data warehouses for easy retrieval.

Lighter (2011) has provided clinically relevant examples using Donabedian's model. Specifically, structure measures describe the facilities, staff, and culture of an organization (e.g., number of licensed beds). Process measures relate to the interface between the patient and the provider (e.g., patient satisfaction). Finally, outcome measures are associated with the efficiency and effectiveness of processes, both clinical and business. Accrediting agencies such as The Joint Commission and the Centers for Medicare and Medicaid Services have developed standards and measures using Donabedian's model that demonstrate desirable characteristics such as importance, scientific soundness, and feasibility.

As projects are developed and implemented, keeping the Donabedian model in mind can help team members analyze the value of projects and link it to information systems. Additionally, with the publication of the Meaningful Use Final Rule (U.S. Department of Health and Human Services, 2014a), projects can be designed to measure the impact of enrolling patients in the clinical patient portal of the electronic medical record. However, ensuring that the integrity of the data is maintained is a mandate that cannot be overlooked.

▶ Data Integrity, Security, Human Protection, and Use

Health information technology makes it possible for all providers to engage in patient-centered care and to manage care through secure use and sharing of health information. However, maintaining **data integrity**, **security**, and **privacy** is a shared responsibility. It is necessary for all care providers, including students, to receive the necessary education to support safe, secure, and trustworthy practice in the healthcare system. As changes in the care delivery system continue to multiply, it is imperative to consider all of the regulatory and technological changes and any changes that impact practice—including any data that are collected during projects and used to change practice.

Meaningful project planning requires a commitment to both data security and protection of human subjects. This understanding is steered by the sensitivity of the data and the consequences for data compromise. Despite precautions, cybercrime continues to rise (Conaty-Buck, 2017). As a quality improvement project or research is executed and data are collected and stored, adhering to the mandates of the Health Insurance Portability and Accountability Act (HIPAA) is essential. This act outlines administrative, physical, and technical safeguards to ensure confidentiality, integrity, and availability of electronic protected health information (U.S. Department of Health and Human Services, 2014b).

Being mindful of data integrity, security, and **human-subject protection** must happen in parallel with measures to address ethical, legal, and security issues. While these issues may be primary responsibilities of the organization as outlined in various organizational policies and position descriptions, the shared responsibility of users of that information cannot be dismissed. Numerous safeguards and processes may be established, but individual responsibility in adhering to and respecting them is the key to maintaining the integrity and protection of data and an individual's privacy.

▶ Summary

- Today's more knowledgeable consumers are demanding accurate and timely data that are easily retrievable and understandable.
- Big data provides a snapshot of what is happening without answering why.
- Small data provides information to answer a specific question and feeds big data by creating knowledge and advancing care.
- Involving IT specialists in projects can lead to more successful projects.
- Linking projects to organizational mission and critical success factors is beneficial in achieving buy-in, support, and sustainment.
- Interprofessional participation in any project is pivotal to success in today's clinical environment, which is characterized by interconnectivity of activities.
- The professional nurse and other members of the healthcare team of the 21st century will be ineffective without a solid foundation and understanding of information technology and competencies.
- Quality and safety initiatives advance organizational value.
- Information exchanges guide decisions and assist in avoiding information security breaches.
- Information systems are the nervous system of meaningful projects.
- Quality, safety, and continuous improvement will be driven by meaningful use processes and the tools necessary to extract data and spread evidence.
- Data and human protection are essential to avoid ethical, legal, and security issues.

Reflection Questions

1. What is the role of nurses, project planners, and interprofessional teams in ensuring projects align healthcare with trends?
2. What are three ways a clinical project may engage stakeholders in moving toward meaningful outcomes?
3. What are the key ways that big and small data are collected and used by organizations?
4. How do these data contribute to a project plan and an organization's plan of action?
5. How might a project planner outline the steps needed to add value-based project outcomes?
6. Why would interprofessional teams and clinical project developers be concerned with the ethical, legal, and human protection of individuals when considering a clinical project?

References

American Association of Colleges of Nursing (AACN). (2006). *The essentials of doctor of nursing educator for professional nursing practice.* Washington, DC: Author.

American Association of Colleges of Nursing (AACN). (2008). *The essentials of baccalaureate education for professional nursing practice.* Washington, DC: Author.

American Association of Colleges of Nursing (AACN). (2011). *The essentials of masters education for professional nursing practice.* Washington, DC: Author.

Ball, M. J., & Douglas, J. V. (1989). Informatics in professional education. *Methods of Information in Medicine, 28*(4), 250–254.

Beal, V. (2014). *Big data.* Retrieved from https://www.webopedia.com/TERM/B/big_data.html

California HealthCare Foundation and First Consulting Group. (2002). *Report identifies positive impact technology can have on nurse productivity and satisfaction.* Retrieved from https://www.chcf.org/press-release /report-identifies-positive-impact-technology-can-have-on-nurse-productivity-and-satisfaction

Cipriano, P. F. (2014). What we measure, we can improve. *The American Nurse.* Retrieved from http:// www.theamericannurse.org/2015/01/05/what-we-measure-we-can-improve

Clark, J., & Lang, N. (1992). Nursing's next advance: An internal classification for nursing practice. *International Nursing Review, 39*(4), 109–111, 128.

Conaty-Buck, S. (2017). Cybersecurity and healthcare records. Tips for ensuring patient safety and privacy. *American Nurse Today, 12*(9), 62–65.

DeLaune, S. C., & Ladner, P. K. (2009)'. *Fundamentals of nursing standards and practice* (3rd ed.). Clifton Park, NY: Delmar Cengage Learning.

Donabedian, A. (1978). The quality of medical care. *Science, 4344,* 856–864.

Fox, S. (2011, February 28). Peer-to-peer health care. *Pew Research Center.* Retrieved from http:// www.pewinternet.org/2011/02/28/peer-to-peer-health-care-2

Gallagher, T. (2012, October 8). The role of informatics in project management. *HIMSS Clinical Informatics Insights.* Retrieved from http://www.himss.org/News/NewsDetail.aspx?ItemNumber =3128

Geibert, R. C. (2017). The information revolution: Using data and technology to support patient care. In S. Davidson, D. Weberg, T. Porter-O'Grady, & K. Malloch (Eds.), *Leadership for evidence-based innovation in nursing and health professions* (pp. 241–262). Burlington, MA: Jones & Bartlett Learning.

Grobe, S. J. (1988). Nursing informatics competencies for nurse educators and researchers. In H. Peterson & U. Gerdin-Jelger (Eds.), *Preparing nurses for using information systems: Recommended informatics competencies.* (pp. 25–40; 117–138 New York, NY: National League for Nursing.

Grobe, S. J. (1989). Nursing informatics competencies. *Methods of Information in Medicine, 28*(4), 267–269.

Healthcare Information and Management Systems Society. (2011, June 17). *Position statement on transforming nursing practice through technology and informatics.* Retrieved from http://www .himss.org/news/transforming-nursing-practice-through-technology-informatics-0

Henly, S. J. (2014). Mother load and mining tools: Big data for science. *Nursing Research, 63*(3), 155.

Institute of Medicine (IOM). (2001). *Crossing the quality chasm: A new health system for the 21st century.* Washington, DC: National Academies Press.

Institute of Medicine (IOM). (2003). *Health professionals education.* Washington, DC: National Academies Press.

Institute of Medicine (IOM). (2011). *The future of nursing: Leading change, advancing health.* Washington, DC: National Academies Press.

Kelly, P. (2012). *Nursing leadership and management* (3rd ed.). Clifton Park, NY: Delmar.

Lewis, A. (2011, November 8). Project management. Part II: What works in nursing informatics? *Advance Web.* Retrieved from http://community.advanceweb.com/blogs/nurses_18/archive/2011/11/08 /project-management-part-ii-what-works-in-nursing-informatics.aspx

Lewis, J. P. (2011). *Project planning, scheduling and control: The ultimate hands-on guide to bridging projects in on time and on budget* (5th ed.). New York, NY: McGraw-Hill.

Lighter, D. M. (2011). *Advanced performance improvement in health care.* Sudbury, MA: Jones & Bartlett Learning.

McCartney, P. R. (2015). Big data science. *The American Journal of Maternal/Child Nursing, 40*(2), 130.

Morrison, I. (2011). *Leading change in health care.* Chicago, IL: AHA Press Health Forum.

National Advisory Council on Nurse Education and Practice. (1997). *Report to the Secretary of the Department of Health and Human Services: A national informatics agenda for nursing education and practice.* Washington, DC: Health Resources and Services Administration.

Nelson, E. C., Batalden, P. B., & Godfrey, M. M. (2007). *Quality by design: A clinical microsystems approach.* San Francisco, CA: Jossey-Bass.

Porter-O'Grady, T., & Malloch, K. (2015). *Quantum leadership: Building better partnerships for sustainable health.* Burlington, MA: Jones & Bartlett Learning.

Shane, B. (2014). *Informatics planning model essential to maximize the effectiveness of IT in supporting program goals.* Retrieved from http://www.bpcgallery.com/informatics_planning.htm

Sicotte, C., & Paré, G. (2010). Success in health information exchange: Solving the implementation puzzle. *Social Science & Medicine, 8*(70), 1159–1165.

Stevens, K. R., & Staley, J. M. (2006). The quality chasm reports, evidence-based practice, and nursing response to improve healthcare. *Nursing Outlook, 54*(2), 94–101.

U.S. Department of Health and Human Services. (2014a). 42 CRF Part 495. *Federal Register, 79* (171).

U.S. Department of Health and Human Services. (2014b). *FY 2014 HHS agency financial report.* Retrieved from https://www.hhs.gov/sites/default/files/afr/fy2014-agency-financial-report-final.pdf

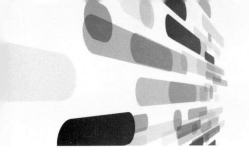

Case Exemplars

▶ Case Study 1

Information Technology: A Valuable Asset for Nursing Informatics Projects

Todd Harlan

As technology has evolved, so has nursing informatics. As a leader of an informatics program preparing master's and doctoral nursing students, an overarching theme is coaching students to strengthen their skill sets for success within the industry and organizations. As students matriculate nationally through informatics tracks, project plans and products must be developed that are based on need and evidence to address constantly changing care needs. Outcomes from the developed products will be evaluated both directly and indirectly, as patient care processes are improved and their sustainable value is realized economically.

Students engage in a series of purposeful activities during the process of selecting improvement projects. An informatics needs assessment is central to understanding needs in all organizations, whether at the micro-, meso-, or macrolevel. The assessment findings require validation, and teams are often used to perform this task. Of note, more interprofessional team validation of findings has become commonplace with the advent of the electronic medical record (EMR), as it crosses all disciplines. The improvement project plan is then developed based on the assessment findings, industry standards, best available evidence, and stakeholder engagement. Students seek and attain approval prior to progressing with any project, including institutional review board (IRB) approvals. Throughout the process, venues are abundant for additional student knowledge attainment and synergy of stakeholders as the plan matures and informatics products are created and implemented.

According to McGonigle and Mastrian (2015), the time interval between conduct of research, project outcome dissemination, and clinical translation can be significant. Both patient and system outcomes may be affected adversely by such delays. The issue within many organizations is translating the data that are embedded within the EMR and trying to extrapolate that information for improved patient outcomes.

During their tenure as informatics program leaders, several students have collaboratively developed systems that support an infrastructure aimed at ensuring quality and safety. One example of a value-based collaborative project is a computerized provider order entry (CPOE) system. Such systems allow physicians to capture order information and access other materials that can improve the overall delivery of care and improve patient outcomes. The Healthcare Information Technology for Economic and Clinical Health (HITECH) provision of the American Recovery and Reinvestment Act provided the supporting rationale for the project. This act provides funding to assist with the development of a health information technology infrastructure that subsequently improves quality and healthcare safety (Radley et al., 2012). Among the provisions noted were incentive payments to physicians and healthcare facilities to support health IT, including CPOE implementation.

While the CPOE example was specific to one discipline's actions, other projects have focused on issues that directly affect patient care and outcomes. Regardless of the IT project, students tend to identify that the task can be daunting and in some cases very difficult to implement. The constantly changing healthcare landscape, reimbursement issues, and accreditation mandates will require easily extractable data for project success. All student projects are vital to the overall knowledge gained within the theory portions of the informatics track. For the primary instructor, ensuring that students are attaining the stated learning objectives and are assigned to knowledgeable preceptors is essential for success.

Nursing informatics will continue to emerge as a dynamic and value-added asset as care delivery shifts to community settings. The development of integrated IT systems will only expand in the coordination of healthcare delivery. Nurses are in pivotal positions to address this call to action.

Reflection Questions

1. When assessing the process of an improvement project, what is a central requirement that is crucial to the success of the project? Describe this process, and discuss the advantages and disadvantages if it is not followed.
2. Discuss the premise of data research and dissemination, and explain how the time between these two phases can affect desired outcomes.
3. As discussed in the case study, computerized provider order entry offers many advantages to physicians and other healthcare providers. Expand on these advantages; also discuss any disadvantages that may exist and be constraints to progress.

References

McGonigle, D., & Mastrian, K. (2015). *Nursing informatics and the foundation of knowledge* (3rd ed.). Burlington, MA: Jones & Bartlett Learning.

Radley, D., Wasserman, M., Olsho, L., Shoemaker, S., Spranca, M., & Bradshaw, B. (2012). Reduction in medication errors in hospitals due to adoption of computerized provider order entry systems. *Journal of the Medical Informatics Association, 20*(3), 470–476. doi:10.1136/2012-001241

▶ Case Study 2

Increasing Nurse Awareness When Administering Medications: The Creation of a Dashboard Warning System

Amy Campbell

Problem Statement

The Institute of Medicine has identified medication errors as being a significant problem causing over 400,000 serious injuries and between 48,000 and 98,000 deaths yearly (Institute of Medicine, 1999). Medication errors are defined by the Agency for Healthcare Research and Quality (AHRQ) as being any discrepancy in the medication dispensing process from pharmacy handling to the nurse administering the medication. A distracted nurse is at a higher risk for committing an error. In the complex healthcare environment where there are bells, warnings, and alerts everywhere, a central question remains: How can the nurse increase awareness before administering medications and avoid additional warning fatigue?

Knowledge Gap

How can a nurse be warned that he or she is at risk for committing an error without adding to the nurse's workload or indirectly causing more distraction?

Project Process and Evaluation Methods

A review of the literature on medication errors was completed to identify multiple causes and contributing factors in medication errors. Six main themes of errors were identified as the most common for affecting the nurse and increasing the risk for medication error: (1) working more than 40 hours a week, (2) large medication loads, (3) large patient loads, (4) large task loads, (5) interruptions, and (6) patient acuity. Quality improvement (QI) projects such as "quiet spaces," staffing changes, and modified scheduling were met with mild to moderate success in reducing errors, but old habits and rising healthcare costs mitigated the long-term success of these changes.

A workflow analysis of a medical-surgical/oncology floor found that nurses were often multitasking while working and were frequently interrupted during documentation and direct patient care by call-lights. The manager worked to maintain a maximum patient–nurse ratio of 1:6 and to schedule staff for no more than 3 days on before giving them 2 days off. A review of documentation revealed that data pertaining to the six identified factors were being gathered and stored in the hospital databases.

Stakeholders comprised of the manager, QI team, information technology (IT) team, clinical analyst team, and leadership sponsor met with the doctor of nursing practice (DNP) student to review the problem, clearly define the scope of the project, and identify barriers and potential solutions to improve the project's success. Additional considerations related to the hospital's limited resources were also addressed. Institutional review board (IRB) and administration approval were obtained as part of the planning process.

A pre-post survey on patient safety was chosen to give to the nursing staff before the dashboard implementation and 30 days following. Data pertaining to the six risk factors were then harvested from the hospital databases for a 60-day period.

The data were organized in order to match each patient's data risk factors (number of times patient used the call-light, number of medications ordered for the patient, sepsis score, etc.) with the nurse who was providing care for that patient. The nurse's lack of situational awareness while administering medications was measured by the number of near-misses (NM) the nurse committed when scanning the wrong patient, wrong medication, or wrong dose or tried to administer a medication in the wrong time frame using a bar-code medication administration system (BCMA). The time frame for when the NM occurred and the nurse's current workload, patient acuity, and level of distraction in relation to the six risk factors were aligned.

An analysis of the historical data found that while not all six factors affected each nurse, at least one or two of the six influenced most nurses negatively. NM thresholds were then determined by the potential risk each factor had on each nurse. After speaking with the nursing staff and the manager, a dashboard design was created that allowed each nurse currently working to quickly visualize both his or her own NM risk level and that of peers using a stoplight color-coded system. The dashboard also identified which of the six factors were currently influencing each nurse's increased risk, allowing for the nurses to make personal modifications to their workflow and allowing for their peers to know how and when to offer assistance. The dashboard was placed within the same room as the automated medication dispensing system so that it would be easily visualized as nurses were getting ready to secure medications for their patient. During the 30-day implementation of the dashboard, NMs were reduced by 15.6%. The postimplementation survey suggested that the dashboard not only improved overall teamwork by 13%, with significant changes specifically noted in the area of respect for team, but also revealed a positive increase in 9 of the 12 patient safety culture areas measured, including a 37% increase in nursing perceived overall patient safety and a 119% increase in frequency of error reporting. As an indirect result of improved teamwork, the average length of stay and discharge turnaround were both reduced. Results were presented to management, and two additional full-time employees were added to the unit to help reduce workload levels and NM risks.

Reflection Questions

1. What are the benefits of identifying causative factors for near-miss medication errors?
2. What role can members of an interprofessional project team play in developing a project to eliminate medication errors?

References

Institute of Medicine (IOM). (1999). *To err is human: Building a safer health system*. Washington, DC: National Academies Press.

CHAPTER 12

Developing Metrics That Support Project Plans, Interventions, and Programs

Patricia L. Thomas

©Shuoshu/DigitalVision Vectors/Getty Images.

ROLES

Communicator   Integrator
Decision-maker   Leader
Information manager

PROFESSIONAL VALUES

Altruism   Social justice
Integrity

CORE COMPETENCIES

Analyzing   Design
Assessment   Interpersonal influence
Coordination   Presenting
Critical thinking   Systems thinking
Data management

▶ Introduction

At its core, the act of "measurement" is fundamentally about communicating change. The more structured and clear the communication, the more likely the change will be accepted, supported, sustained, and replicated (Datsenko & Schenk, 2013). Communication can take many forms, ranging from large national impact through academic, peer-reviewed journal publications to local demonstrations within single inpatient units using dashboards, posted charts, and/or graphs. Regardless of scale and audience, in today's U.S. healthcare system, one of the most important stories to tell is that of performance optimization and, more broadly, that of quality imporvement. These initiatives represent central strategies for improving the value proposition of an oft fragmented and inefficient care delivery system (Radnor, Holweg, & Waring, 2012).

Predicated on the Institute of Medicine reports *To Err Is Human: Building a Safer Health System* (1999), *Crossing the Quality Chasm: A New Health System for the 21st Century* (2001), and *Health Professions Education: A Bridge to Quality* (2003), several national imperatives were established. One of the most widely accepted was the Institute on Healthcare Improvements strategy and model created as a framework to discipline improvement work and foster replication of initiatives directed toward patient safety and quality improvement (Insititute for Healthcare Improvement [IHI], 2015a). Based on elements from these activities, a three-step process to guide improvement work has been established: (1) Identify problems or opportunities for improvement, (2) select appropriate measures of these areas, and (3) obtain a baseline assessment of current practices and then remeasure to assess the effect of improvement efforts on measured performance as foundational managing projects within health delivery. The discussion within this chapter focuses on the second of these steps—*how*

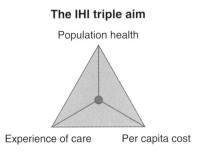

FIGURE 12-1 The IHI Triple Aim

The IHI Triple Aim framework was developed by the Institute for Healthcare Improvement in Boston, Massachusetts (www.ihi.org).

to select the right measures for a project or program and the influence of organizational decision-making, culture, and evidence-based practices.

While many examples of healthcare quality improvement frameworks exist in the literature, one of the simplest and most popular is known as the Triple Aim, developed by the IHI (2015b), as illustrated in **FIGURE 12-1**. The framework suggests that in order to build lasting and meaningful change, new initiatives must be developed to communicate three sides of the same story:

1. The patient experience of care (including quality and satisfaction)
2. The health of populations
3. The cost of health care

To be successful, the story of a performance optimization project or program, told through the lens of data, must include a chapter from all three. The goal here is to provide simple, actionable instructions on how to weave together that story using data. Recently, efforts have been under way to establish the quadruple aim to highlight satisfaction with work life for healthcare workers. Realizing the experience and impact of clinician burnout, turnover, and disengagement of employees and patient safety, the quadruple aim seeks to highlight how members of a team delivering care influence outcomes. Measurement of employee satisfaction, employee engagement, and staff retention or turnover could provide metrics in support of this aim (Bodenheimer & Sinsky, 2014).

▶ Organizational Culture and Project Management

While the discipline of project management framed by data is critical to project or program success, the culture within an organization or unit cannot be ignored. In recent years, recognition for both the "soft" and "hard" sides of leadership and project management have been recognized, in large part because projects or programs failed (Radnor et al., 2012; Sheppy, Zuliani, & Mclntosh, 2012). Malloch and Porter-O'Grady (2010); Melnyk and Fineout-Overholt (2015); and Nelson, Batalden, and Godfrey (2007) address organizational culture and change leadership as foundational to implementation of evidence-based practices and quality improvement, emphasizing the need to honestly assess the environment to leverage strengths (and champions) and prepare for resistance or compliance proactively.

Common barriers to successful implementation of projects or their replication are lack of leader champions, insufficient human and fiscal resources, and unrealistic expectations regarding the time necessary for design and achieving desired outcomes. Schein (2004) describes organizational culture and leadership as two sides of the same coin with both having the significant influence within organizations, particularly when instituting change. Inclusive of the spoken and unspoken values, norms, and espoused beliefs, awareness of the culture is essential to success but is often overlooked at the start of a program or project. Setting project goals and developing a charter for the work team that outlines expectations, timelines, and lines of accountability and authority structure expectations is an initial step. What is often missed is the discussion and planning directed toward perceptions, change leadership strategies, and methods to address the team activities that will be undertaken if the agreed-upon changes start to backslide to the previous state. Each of these has distinct strategies for management and requires acknowledgment of the power that culture has in influencing them (Andre & Sjovold, 2017; Shirley, 2011)

Lam and Robertson (2012) were curious about the ways organizational culture was attributed to the success or failure of improvement projects without empiric support for this attribution. They developed and administered a survey to 1,027 healthcare employees to investigate perceptions of organizations' culture and willingness to participate in continuous improvement projects. Experience and participation in previous improvement projects, tenure, and organizational demonstration of supporting change had a statistically significant influence on individuals' willingness to participate in improvement projects. The use of a disciplined project management structure versus ad hoc project management did not have a significant influence. The results highlighted that an organization's support and success in implementing change greatly influenced willingness to participate in improvement projects, thus becoming a part of the culture.

The link to organizational readiness and assessment of this readiness, including data availability, administrative support, and outcome analyst support, provide organizational information to determine how poised a team is to accept change. The rationale for a change readiness assessment or evaluation of the culture provides important information to leaders that can reduce or eliminate impacts on staffing and caregivers who will be affected by a project (Brown & Hough-Falk, 2014).

▶ Use of Evidence-Based Practice: An Intertwined Element

Evidence-based practice and evidence-based medicine are established "buzzwords" that get affirmative nods from many practitioners across disciplinary lines. Despite this affirmation, many disciplines have been slow to adopt evidence-based practices and often identify solutions to problems or new changes to implement without the benefit of evidence. For discussions related to the selection of metrics, project development, and the ensuing evaluation and alignment to evidence in the design of the program or project aims and in the development of activities or interventions, is essential (Malloch & Porter-O'Grady, 2010; Nelson et al., 2007). Without clarity derived from definitions and reputable evidence found in the literature, selection of interventions based on levels of evidence acceptable in the scope of the change (or project), replication is difficult, and credibility of outcomes is questioned (Hall & Roussel, 2014; Melnyk & Fineout-Overholt, 2015). While outside the focus of this chapter, understanding the model an organization has selected to evaluate evidence and the framework used to implement evidence are important considerations for the project manager to explore during the predesign work.

Levels of evidence have been established and are generally accepted across the country. Often depicted in a pyramid, evidence at the lowest and widest point includes animal research, followed in each level by case studies or reports, case control studies, cohort studies, randomized controlled trials, systematic reviews, and topped with metanalysis at the top of the pyramid (Hall & Roussel, 2014). Evidence is often described by its strength, with expert opinion, experience, theory, and qualitative studies having least strength and again moving through a pyramid structure with non-experimental studies, research studies or randomized controlled studies, and evidence studies as categories reaching the top of the pyramid. Inherent in this evaluation of strength are components of consistency, quantity, and quality of the evidence (Melnyk & Fineout-Overholt, 2015). It is incumbent on the project manager and members of the team to consider levels and strength of evidence using structures and processes within the organization as projects are designed and progress. Depending on the project or program undertaken, the evidence base that underpins the work may determine the metrics and measures of success.

▶ The Cost/Quality Dance

In this era of healthcare reform, ignoring costs is both outdated and detrimental. Irrespective of the team composition, demonstrating a positive impact to the financial landscape in an organization often distinguishes work that will continue versus work or workstreams slated for elimination. Gone are the days when quality reigned as the single driver of clinical success. What is now recognized is that efficiency, effectiveness, and awareness of cost support improvement in quality and clinical outcomes.

Several terms related to costs are regularly used, so it is important for project managers and team members to establish where the project resides in relation to the cost-quality equation. Caution needs to be used when discussing cost because there are times when spending money or having a higher cost can be advantageous if the clinical care outcomes are improved and consistent. Significant healthcare expenditures are made on duplicative care, readmissions, and incomplete care. Therefore, consultation with financial analysts and individuals with a systems lens to examine upstream and downstream impacts is key.

▶ Cost Avoidance, Cost-Effectiveness, and Cost Benefit

When establishing a financial impact, defining terms for both team members and stakeholders is needed. When engaged in change work, it is common to assume that the driver for the project rests in cost reduction, often translated as job loss. Project managers have an important leadership responsibility in reducing the stress and fear of a team so that creative and innovative solutions can be formulated. *Cost avoidance* is defined as costs in the future that will not be incurred because of a change in practice or process. Think of this like you would think of preventative maintenance on your car. Often you have a cost in the short-run (like an oil change), but you avoid blowing your head gasket. The same holds true in health care. If we spend money on this now, we could avoid expenses (and potentially negative health outcomes). Some view this kind of savings as a "soft saving" because you have not spent the money yet, and other factors could arise that negate the savings.

Cost-effectiveness analysis is often used to highlight areas where resources could be used differently to achieve a desired effect. It showcases opportunities to employ inexpensive interventions that have the potential to reduce disease burden, achieve outcomes, and reduce expense. An example of this would be oral rehydration for children with diarrhea. More than 1 million children die from dehydration annually. While oral rehydration does not decrease the incidence of diarrhea in children, it can reduce the severity and mortality associated with it. The cost of the oral rehydration pales in comparison to the hospitalization costs and critical care expenses associated with childhood diarrhea. *Cost-benefit analysis* assigns a dollar valued on both the cost and the effectiveness of an intervention, recognizing individual and societal benefits that often influence policy and decision-makers. An example of this would be purchasing lift equipment to void employee injuries, recognizing it will take time to pay for the equipment, but by having fewer employees injured during lift or transfer, the equipment will pay for itself because of the money saved on lost time from work, workers' compensation costs, and overtime. A project manager would need to keep the potential or desired financial impact in view for the teams he or she leads. Often, a member of the finance department will be a member of the project team or will serve as a consultant to the team so that financial analysis is based on the design and development of each specific project.

▶ Selecting the Right Variables to Tell Your Story

Selecting variables to establish measures of progress and success can be daunting. Members of the project team often come from different disciplines, educational programs, and job or role expectations, bringing diversity and a wide space for misunderstandings. As the project manager, one of the roles will be to simplify the process and bring a sense of confidence and inclusion to those completing work. To that end, using metaphors that bring common meaning and understanding to others offers a space for shared learning and understanding. When discussing **metrics**, measures, and variables, a helpful metaphor for groups that will implement change is that of "telling a story through data." What follows is an example of how "telling a story" can guide variable selection and bring clarity around complex topics.

Take a look at any home library. The shelves are, most likely, a cornucopia of different genres of books. The subjects could range from science fiction and biographies to poetry and romance. Each tells a unique story from a unique perspective, with a unique cast of characters. So is the case in health care—there are many unique stories to be told, each with its own unique storytelling style and supporting cast of characters. These stories can be told through the lens of data and measurement. Think of each chart, graph, and dashboard as a chapter of the story being told. Each measure or variable is a different character, with a specific role and perspective. The Agency for Healthcare Research and Quality (AHRQ) defines three general story genres, each with its own matching style and measurement purpose: (1) quality improvement, (2) accountability, and (3) research (AHRQ, 2014).

Quality Improvement

Measures of clinical quality improvement can be used to illustrate practices within or across an organization and also could apply to smaller groups such as units or service lines. These measures cover many aspects of patient care such as health outcomes, patient safety, care coordination, or adherence to clinical guidelines. One of the simplest examples of a health outcome measure is 30-day mortality rate. Another example is the percentage of patients age 65 years and older with a body mass index (BMI) greater than or equal to 23. The resulting value is reflective of the quality of clinical service being delivered to the patient population.

▶ Accountability

Measures of accountability support the needs of audiences other than those that directly provide care, such as payers, regulators, accrediting organizations, or patients. The results are used to compare provider groups, select providers based on performance, or establish a case for providing financial rewards (AHRQ, 2014). One example of a measure of accountability is the percentage of advanced practice registered nurses (such as certified nurse–midwives) in a given service line (OB/GYN, for example). This is a measure of nursing quality and professional development within a specified service line and could be used by the department to make decisions about nurses' pay scales.

Research

Measures for use in clinical research differ from quality improvement and accountability measures by their intended use. The primary use of measures in research is to generate new knowledge that is generalizable (AHRQ, 2014). These insights are valuable in setting health policy, evaluating programs, or assessing the effectiveness of a clinical practice or guideline, typically requiring larger sample sizes and more detailed data collection. Very often, the collection of data for use in clinical research will require the engagement of an institutional review board (IRB) to enforce ethical or patient safety guidelines.

▶ Fundamental Types of Measures

Process Measures

Measures of clinical process describe "activities carried out by healthcare workers to deliver services" (AHRQ, 2014). Measures of this type reflect specific and observable aspects of clinical practice. A prominent example comes from emergency cardiac care. For patients presenting to the emergency department with STEMI (ST-segment elevation myocardial infarction), door-to-balloon time measures a process that starts with the patient's arrival and ends with intervention in the cardiac catheterization laboratory. This is a process measure that describes the total time necessary to complete a series of processes associated with treating a patient with STEMI, performed by multiple care team members. A key feature of process measures is that they can be easily and clearly defined. As a result, when properly defined, process measures are generally not case-mix or risk-adjusted.

Information about completed processes emerges from two sources. First, the process can be directly observed. Staff with a stopwatch can time how long it takes to complete a specific task or shadow clinicians to ensure a specific task is completed or not. This is referred to as upstream measurement—the measurement is taken *as the action is being completed*. One example is the observational audit of staff to ensure that the proper hand-washing procedure is followed.

On the other hand, downstream measurement is generated from information on processes that *have already been completed*. Here, data are often extracted from administrative sources such as patient charts or the electronic medical record. Door-to-balloon time for STEMI patients is an example of downstream measurement because the measure is reported as the sum of the time it takes to complete multiple processes and therefore is typically extracted from the medical record after the sample population of patients has been discharged. Another example is the examination of a patient charts to see if fall prevention education was delivered. The chart review takes place after the process of delivering fall prevention education has been completed.

Downstream measures have two important limitations that cannot be overlooked. First, downstream measures typically only indicate whether or not a process was completed; they are binary indicators, lacking any qualifiers. They do not clearly indicate *how* the process was completed. Expanding on the example of fall prevention education, using a downstream measure for this process would not reveal any information about how much time was taken to speak to the patient and gives no indication that the patient fully comprehended the information provided, two pieces of information that could be captured if the process had been directly observed. Second, downstream measurement introduces recall bias by relying on staff to record information after the task has been completed, sometimes several hours later. For these reasons, upstream measurement is the preferred option where available but should be balanced against the greater demands placed on the cost of gathering this data (such as staff time and expense).

Outcome Measures

Although representing different viewpoints, both measures of process and measures of outcomes must be included to tell the complete story of any project or program. Outcome measures are the cornerstone of quality improvement. For many projects and programs, improving patient outcomes is the final goal. Outcomes capture a variety of health states such as mortality, physiologic measures (blood pressure, laboratory test results), and patient-reported health status (functional status and symptoms) (AHRQ, 2014). These variables represent final goals of clinical interventions and processes—improved health status for patients or populations.

Process measures and outcomes measures are intrinsically linked. One of the most common mistakes made in measurement strategy is the conflation of the two. Evaluating a care management training program on medication reconciliation in primary care practices represents two things. First are the process measures derived from the training process. Second are the outcomes or results of this training on medication reconciliation as the outcome. It is not uncommon for these distinct measures to be described as one entity. In developing a project or program, calling out the distinctions between process and outcomes is essential so that measurement and clarity around accountability and results can be determined.

Qualitative Measures

While quantitative measurement is most commonly used based on specificity and ease in data gathering and analysis, qualitative measurement offers a different perspective. Measures that tell the story of a stakeholder's opinion about a process are called qualitative measures because they convey deeper meaning regarding quality, or how *well* a given process was fulfilled. A plethora of qualitative measures can be found on the Hospital Consumer Assessment of Healthcare Providers and Systems, or HCAHPS, survey (also known as the CAHPS Hospital Survey). HCAHPS is a national, standardized, publicly reported survey of patient perceptions of care received during a hospitalization (Centers for Medicare and Medicaid Services [CMS], 2014). It is a 27-question survey about a patient's recent hospital stay, taken from a random, monthly sample of all eligible discharges. One example qualitative measure from this survey tool is the percentage of patients who report that their nurses "always" communicated well during their stay (H-COMP-1-A-P). This measure is considered to be qualitative because it reflects a person's opinion about nurse communication— what is considered to be "good" or "effective" communication varies from person to person. Similar surveys exist for home and hospice care (HHCAPS).

▶ Selecting the Right Data

When possible, measure sets are best focused on the patient or individual, commonly referred to as "patient-centric." This means that when read together, the measures show how a patient or population of patients progresses through a given process or disease state. This simplifies understanding and provides a platform for replication.

Matching Populations

When selecting sets of variables, care should be taken to represent the same time frame and the same target population across the entire set. Mismatches of this type are common. Using **TABLE 12-1** as a reference, there would be little insight to be gained by reporting the average length of stay for a population of patients discharged between the months of January to June at the same time as 30-day all-cause mortality rate for patients discharged between the months of July and December. By definition, these are two different populations with two different stories to tell. This noise makes interpreting any trend, change, or intervention outcome difficult or even impossible to discern. In addition to reporting time frames, other mismatches can arise in the underlying population (different groups of patients) and processes without connection or causal relationship. Drawing conclusions about the impact a change has when the "noise" is not accounted for can lead to attribution that is distorted or inaccurate.

TABLE 12-1 Sample Inpatient Heart Failure Measure Set

Variable Description	Data Source	Measure Type
Heart Failure & Shock with Major Complications (MS-DRG 291)	CMS (ICD-10-CM)	Outcome; quantitative
Heart Failure & Shock with Complications (MS-DRG 292)	CMS (ICD-10-CM)	Outcome; quantitative
Heart Failure and Shock Without Complications or Major Complications (MS-DRG 293)	CMS (ICD-10-CM)	Outcome; quantitative
Average Length of Stay (ALOS)	Administrative clinical data; EMR	Process; quantitative
30-Day, All-Cause Mortality Rate	Administrative clinical data; EMR	Outcome; quantitative
Patients Discharged to Ambulatory Care or Home Health Care	Administrative clinical data; EMR	Process; quantitative
30-Day, All-Cause Unplanned Readmission Rate	Administrative clinical data; EMR	Outcome; quantitative
Patients Who Received Heart Failure Education	Administrative clinical data; EMR	Process; quantitative

Common Data Sources

- CMS
- National Database of Nursing Quality Indicators (NDNQI)
- AHRQ National Quality Measures Clearinghouse
- Healthcare Effectiveness Data and Information Set (HEDIS)
- Organizational administrative and claims data

Benefits of Using Established Measures

Many of us are tempted to write or establish individual data definitions as a means to highlight the uniqueness of an organization or a patient population. This can be initiated because individuals recognize that the current available data are valued by those engaged in the project or data that are readily available. Oftentimes, individuals look for ways to stimulate "buy-in," particularly when the "charge" or expectation to make meaningful change originates outside the work team expected to generate the change. While tempting, this undertaking requires knowledge and analysis not generally found in healthcare organizations and should be avoided if established national or specialty-specific data definitions exist. Over the last decade, significant progress has been made in establishing evidence-based, validated, credible data definitions that promote comparability within a single facility or to other organizations, especially when participating in regional or national quality improvement collaboratives.

Eliminating Unnecessary Measures

In Lean and Project Management Book of Knowledge (PMBOK) methodology, any work that adds cost, time, or expands the scope of this work without also adding value is considered to be wasteful. One specific type of waste that is applicable to measurement strategy is called overprocessing. Overprocessing can take many forms, including requesting and processing more information than is necessary or information that will never be used, or reporting duplicative information (Hadfield, Holmes, Kozlowski, Sperl, & Tapping, 2012). A central tenet of Lean is to only measure that which one intends to impact through a project or program. Eliminating waste from your dashboard—in the form of vestigial or unnecessary variables—will increase the clarity and impact of the story being told therein. Additionally, and perhaps more importantly, it will increase the ability to glean new knowledge such as trends from the data, which could otherwise be hidden behind the noise of unnecessary measures. For example, if the goal of a program is to establish a process for complex care coordination in the emergency department (ED), the measurement of ED median arrival-to-discharge time adds no valuable information.

To eliminate waste from an established dashboard of measures, begin by clarifying the reporting and communication needs of involved stakeholders. Look for measures which do not include information which is being expressly requested. This step is also a centerpiece of change management—if stakeholders are not involved early in the process of making changes, there is a higher risk that disruptions could arise further on.

▶ Data Management Plan

No matter what program or project is going to be evaluated, a data management plan should be developed to help guide the process of selecting the appropriate **metrics**. Using a structured approach provides a proactive guide to ensure the best measurement is initially identified and that all of the information needed for evaluation is obtained. There are six basic steps to follow, which are (1) define data needs, (2) identify data sources, (3) identify performance measures, (4) design the study, (5) retrieve the data, and (6) analyze the data.

Step One: Define Data Needs

Defining necessary data depends upon the questions to be answered. There are two general types of questions. First are quantitative questions such as "Who?" "What?" and "How many?" These questions generate numerical data that can be counted, ranked, and statistically analyzed, such as volume and frequency data. Quantitative questions are generally asked to verify something or make a prediction (Shank, 2006). Calculated means or averages can be trended over time. Medians, or the middle point of data sets, are better to use for data sets with extreme values (Brown, Aydin, & Donaldson, 2008; Geary & Clanton, 2011).

The second type of question, qualitative, seeks to answer "Why?" "Why not?" and "How?" These questions are open ended to generate lots of information and gain a deeper understanding of the issue being studied. Analysis of qualitative responses is done by reviewing the responses and identifying any common themes. Qualitative questions are not as frequently used in hospitals but can often give you more timely data and be less expensive to generate (Geary & Clanton, 2011; Hoff & Sutcliffe, 2006).

Using both quantitative and qualitative questions can result in a measurement set that more thoroughly evaluates a process or program. The patient satisfaction surveys used by most hospitals include both quantitative and qualitative questions. Quantitative questions ask patients to rank their response on some sort of numerical scale and address items such as level of satisfaction with nursing care, discharge planning, pain management, environmental cleanliness, and quality of food. These data can be compared and trended over time to include previous information. Most surveys also have open-ended questions that assess patients' opinions or comments. When specific comments are recurrent, then trends can be identified. Qualitative information can direct how an aspect of care might be improved or identify processes that can be replicated. Using both quantitative and qualitative data provides a holistic approach to any type of evaluation and should be used whenever possible (Geary & Clanton, 2011).

Two quality-control tools that are useful in determining a specific type of questions and measurements needed for program evaluation are process flowcharts and cause-and-effect diagrams. Process flow diagrams provide a visualization of all of the steps and decision points involved in a process. The first step in creating a flow diagram is to identify the beginning and the end point of the process. An oval shape is used to represent these points. Hospital processes are usually very complex, so it is important to establish exactly what part of the process is being reviewed. The different steps within a process are represented by rectangles and appear in the order as they occur in the process. All processes have decision points that are represented in a flow diagram as diamonds. The different answers at these decision points will either lead to the next step in the process or outside the process where some other step or decision must be made before the process can continue. The number of decision points contained in a process is an indication of the process complexity. The more complex the process is, the greater the chance for breakdown or undesired outcomes (Geary & Clanton, 2011).

Key measurements for analysis can be identified by reviewing the flowchart key process steps and decision points (Geary & Clanton, 2011; Okes & Westcott, 2001; Wescott, 2013). For example, flow diagrams can identify missing, redundant, or erroneous steps and point to improvement actions. An example of a flow diagram is shown in **FIGURE 12-2**.

A cause-and-effect diagram is useful in demonstrating the many different contributing causes of a particular problem. To construct this type of diagram, the problem (effect) is noted in the box at the right side of the chart, and then major categories and subcategories that identify possible different causes are listed. Typical categories when discussing patient care problems are patient factors, staff factors, physician factors, administrative factors (policies and procedures), environmental factors, and equipment factors. A benefit of creating a cause-and-effect diagram is the brainstorming of all possible factors, which yields a broad range of possible measurements, ensuring a thorough review. The cause-and-effect diagram shown in

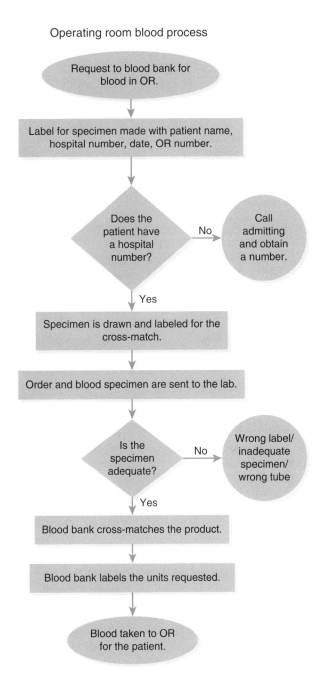

FIGURE 12-2 Process Flow Diagram

FIGURE 12-3 is a continuation of Figure 12-2 (Geary & Clanton, 2011, p. 129). After reviewing the process flow, the step of cross-matching the patient's blood specimen was identified as being a common cause for the delay. A cause-and-effect diagram was constructed to illustrate all of the possible reasons why a problem with blood cross-matching might occur (Geary & Clanton, 2011).

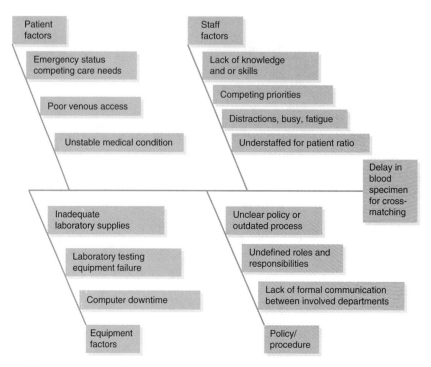

FIGURE 12-3 Cause-and-effect Diagram

Step Two: Identify Data Sources

Hospitals today, more than ever, collect a large amount of data. Much of what hospitals measure is required by the CMS to receive reimbursement for services or by The Joint Commission to demonstrate compliance with accreditation standards. The Joint Commission Hospital Standards require hospitals to collect data to monitor performance pertaining to restraint use, moderate sedation, adverse drug reactions, medication errors, results of resuscitation, use of blood products, procedure complications, and preoperative and postoperative diagnosis discrepancies (The Joint Commission, 2017). Hospitals also have ongoing measurements/counts of infection rates, patient falls, mortality, length of patient stay, and other metrics designed to analyze processes of care and productivity of services. In addition to acute care metrics, HEDIS data for population health metrics and community-based care services are gaining prominence.

Many hospitals participate in disease-specific registries such as the Society of Thoracic Surgeons, the American College of Cardiology, and the National Surgical Quality Improvement Program. These national databases have validated measures of risk-adjusted patient outcomes for specific procedures such as coronary artery bypass surgery, percutaneous coronary interventions, and surgical care. The metrics are designed to measure evidence-based physician practices.

The most common direct measure of nursing is the NDNQI. This metric set was developed in 1998 by the American Nurses Association and became part of Press Ganey in 2014 and is used by more than 26,000 organizations in the United States (Press Ganey, 2014, 2017). The NDNQI based on the National Quality Forum–endorsed safe practices. The National Quality Forum's *Safe Practices for*

Better Healthcare was originally released in 2003 and has been updated four times since then to incorporate current evidence and new measures (National Quality Forum, 2010). Of these measures, those most closely linked to nursing practice are referred to as nursing-sensitive measures and include nursing workforce (staffing plan and resource allocation), patient care information, order read-back and abbreviations, labeling of diagnostic studies, discharge systems, medication reconciliation, hand hygiene, surgical site infection prevention, multidrug-resistant organism prevention, venous thrombosis prevention, glycemic control, wrong-site-surgery prevention, pressure ulcer prevalence, patient falls, urinary catheter–associated infections, central line catheter–associated bloodstream infections, and ventilator-associated pneumonia (Geary & Clanton, 2011; National Quality Forum, 2010).

In October 2008, the CMS identified eight hospital-acquired conditions (HAC) that would cause hospitals to lose some of their Medicare reimbursement. This list has been updated regularly to include safe practices and evidence supporting effective preventative measures as the standard of care. Many HACs are specifically linked to nursing care, including stage III or IV pressure ulcers; falls and trauma; catheter-associated urinary tract infections, vascular catheter–associated infections; surgical site infections following heart surgery, bariatric procedures; and spine, neck, shoulder, and elbow procedures and glycemic control. The quality of nursing care also contributes in preventing the other HACs, including foreign object retained after surgery, air embolism, blood incompatibility, and deep vein thrombosis following knee and hip replacements (Geary & Clanton, 2011).

Caution is needed when using the CMS core measures, HAC data, or any data derived from administrative or coded data for analysis or conclusions. Administrative data are generated from patient classification and billing codes. Diagnostic, procedural, and complication codes are determined by medical record reviewers based on what is documented in the medical record according to established coding criteria. Thus, only what is documented in the record and interpreted by the coders will be part of the administrative database. Administrative data is not risk-adjusted for patient condition, does not include any clinical information, and can be misinterpreted in the coding process (Ko, 2009; Missel & Thomas, 2015). This methodology is acknowledged in the analysis (Geary & Clanton, 2011).

Step Three: Identify Performance Measures

Once the topic, specific questions, and data sources have been identified, specific measures are determined. Three types of measures are used, including structural, process, and outcome measures. Structural measures refer to the attributes of a healthcare organization and how it is organized to deliver care. Examples of structural measures include staffing ratios, patient skill mix, and procedure volumes. These measures are typically easy to access from administrative databases and do not require manual data collection. In the past, measuring surgical volumes or specific patient program enrollment volumes has been used as a measure of an organization's quality of care. However, the significance of the relationship between volumes and outcomes has only been demonstrated for a few procedures (Geary & Clanton, 2011; Ko, 2009). Structural measures can be indirectly related to both process and outcome measures. Having a combination of all three types of measures can be useful in evaluating different aspects of a process; these measures are shown in **TABLE 12-2**.

TABLE 12-2 Structure, Process, and Outcome Measures for Cardiac Catheterization

Measure	Jan	Feb	Mar	April	May	June	July	Aug	Sept	Oct	Nov	Dec	Total
Volume (structural measures)													
No. of catheters													
No. of diagnostic													
No. of interventional													
Process measures													
Closure device used (Y/N)													
Fluoro time													
No. of stents													
Complications (outcome measures)													
No. of hematomas													

No. of required transfusions							
No. requiring surgery							
No. requiring unplanned intervention							
No. of acute closures							
No. of closures w/in 6 mos							
No. of codes E—expired; S—survived							
No. of balloon pumps used							
No. of AMI* following catheterization							
No. of deaths							

*AMI, acute myocardial infarction.

Process measures typically evaluate whether processes are being followed as designed. They can measure specific steps of a process or an entire process and usually fall into categories of financial, utilization, compliance, disease specific, and satisfaction with care (Lighter, 2011; Missel & Thomas, 2015). The CMS core measures are all process measures designed to determine the frequency of specific evidence-based practices. The CMS requires measuring processes to facilitate optimal patient outcomes that should occur. The underlying assumption is that if the core measure practices for pneumonia patients, for example, are instituted, then a patient with pneumonia will have a greater chance of having a positive outcome. However, many factors and processes can influence patients' outcomes, so inferences regarding any causal relationships should be made with caution. The patient's other health risks may affect his or her recovery, infection prevention practices of the patient's caregivers could cause the patient to develop a nosocomial infection, and the skill of the cardiologist can determine the success of any cardiac interventions. Therefore, measuring outcomes such as complications, infections, and mortality is also important in the overall evaluation of a program or project (Geary & Clanton, 2011).

Outcome measures are used to determine the effectiveness of processes. Two types of outcomes are common in health care—operational and clinical outcomes. Both are important in program evaluation. Operational outcomes measure how well a nonclinical process is performing and include financial data, environmental inspection data, patient satisfaction with food, and cleanliness. Clinical outcome measures are specific to a clinical condition or the result of specific treatment and care. Many national registries such as the National Surgical Quality Improvement Program provide clinical outcome data that is risk adjusted for each patient according to comorbidities and other identified related factors (Ko, 2009; Missel & Thomas, 2015). Risk-adjusted outcome data are a more accurate measure of how well a treatment or process is working.

There are many valid and reliable assessment tools that can be used to define concepts to be measured. For example, when measuring patients' risk for skin breakdown, using the Braden Scale to define high risk gives a specific definition and ensures an objective, consistent measurement. One should not assume to know the meaning, as many concepts can be subjectively defined. For example, measuring a patient's level of pain will vary from patient to patient and could vary based on what specific type of pain measurement scale is used to quantify the pain. A level-5 pain may be the most severe pain on a 1–5 scale but moderate pain on a 1–10 scale. Another example is the different definitions of fall rates; some include patient and visitor falls while others include only patients. Performance measures must be defined before measuring and preferably using definitions that have already been validated and used in the nursing literature (Geary & Clanton, 2011).

Performance measures need to be reliable and valid. Reliability is defined as the extent to which the data generated are consistent with what is being measured and the variable of interest is measured the same way in each participant (Missel & Thomas, 2015; Polit & Beck, 2004). Performance measures are said to be valid when they measure what is intended to be studied. Poor validity can occur if the measure is indirectly linked to a concept or if the variables are not clearly defined.

Step Four: Design the Study

The study design is determined by the focus of the project or program and the specific aspects being evaluated. However, some basic concepts are defining the population of interest and determining the sample size. For example, if the project focuses on preventing urinary tract infections in hospitalized patients, the population of interest would be all patients who have an indwelling catheter. In a large hospital, it may not be possible to include all patients, so a representative sample would be needed. The current minimum sample size is 5% or 30 items, whichever is greater (Williams & Geary, 1997). If the population is less than 30, every case needs to be reviewed (Geary & Clanton, 2011).

Step Five: Retrieve the Data

Many projects fail because data retrieval is not systematically planned, resulting in wrong or incomplete data being obtained, leading to an inability to analyze or measure the concept of interest (Lighter, 2011; Missel & Thomas, 2015). Systematically planning the retrieval of data includes deciding where and how to access data that are already being collected, or, if data are not already available, deciding who will collect the data, how data will be gathered, and the specific time period for the collection. This is especially critical to do if more than one person is doing the data retrieval to ensure consistent methods. Data collection tools, such as the one shown in **TABLE 12-3** (Geary & Clanton, 2011, pp. 136–138), are helpful in ensuring consistency in data retrieval.

Data can come from a variety of sources and retrieval methods and can include observation, medical record review, surveys, and interviews. The information needed will determine the best source of the data; the more direct measure of a concept, the stronger the analysis. For example, observing a practice is a more accurate measure than reviewing a chart for documentation of the practice. The ease of obtaining data is also an important factor and can sometimes cause one to use a more indirect measure of the concept (Geary & Clanton, 2011).

It is also necessary to decide on the time period for measurement. Most administrative data, such as core measures, are retrospective measurements. Advantages of retrospective data collection include convenience and use of administrative databases, which allow for quick and large-scale evaluations to be done. Examples of retrospective data retrieval include using administrative data based on specific codes, medical record abstractions from previous hospitalizations, and posthospital/procedure surveys. A disadvantage of retrospective data is that there is a delay of sometimes several months between when a process change or improvement action is implemented and when the retrospective data will be available to analyze for any effects. Therefore, retrospective data are not best for projects of an urgent nature needing immediate review.

Concurrent measurement refers to real-time data collection; the length of time for data collection depends on the amount of data needed to reach the appropriate sample size. The disadvantage of concurrent measurement is that it takes more time and effort to collect the data. The advantages, however, are that data can be trended (Geary & Clanton, 2011; Missel & Thomas, 2015).

During this collection time, any issues can be promptly identified and addressed. With retrospective data, any issues have already occurred, and there is no opportunity to intervene at the time of occurrence.

Step Six: Analyze the Data

The last step of the data management plan is to analyze the measurement data to determine any necessary changes. Data analysis is often the weakest step and is frequently inadequately performed. There are some simple statistical tools that can assist in analyzing the effect of an action or the success of a project. Several different

TABLE 12-3 Patient Safety Liaisons Data Collection Form

Patient Safety Unit-Based Rounds
Unit: _____ Month/Year _____ Completed by: _____

Issue—Mark Each as Yes; No; n/a	MR No.	MR No.	MR No.	MR No.	MR No.
Patient Interview and Observation Items:					
1. The patient was encouraged not to leave his/her clinical area and if he/she does, to have signed release in chart.					
2. The correct armband is on the patient.					
3. Ask the patient if new caregivers are asking him/her to state his/her full name and checking his/her armband prior to giving him/her medications or blood.					
4. Patients at a high risk for falling have on a yellow armband and a fall leaf placed on the door.					
Medications/IV solutions					
5. IV medications are labeled with correct patient name, time IV hung, and ordered drug/dose if not already labeled.					
6. The IV site is dated, timed, and changed every 72 hours.					
7. The IV pump library is in use for heparin, insulin, and chemotherapy agents.					
8. A medication reconciliation form is completed on admission.					
9. PCA pumps have a booklet and a warning label for patient to push only.					

Patient Safety Unit-Based Rounds Unit: _____ Month/Year _____ Completed by: _____					
Issue—Mark Each as Yes; No; n/a	MR No.	MR No.	MR No.	MR No.	MR No.
Chart review					
10. Documentation of read-back of orders has been done.					
11. Documentation of read-back of critical values, tests, and procedure results has been done.					
12. Allergies are documented on all required forms.					
13. Signature indicating informed consent has been obtained for any surgical or invasive bedside procedure and matches the procedure on the order or postprocedure note.					
14. All invasive procedures have a final time out entered.					
15. No "do not use" abbreviations are found in the progress notes or orders. If so, list which ones (write "none" or the specific abbreviations used).					
16. The Morse Fall Scale is recorded on the graphics according to the patient's risk level.					
17. The Braden Scale is recorded on the initial assessment sheet according to the patient's risk level.					

(continues)

TABLE 12-3 Patient Safety Liaisons Data Collection Form					*(continued)*
Patient Safety Unit-Based Rounds **Unit:** _____ **Month/Year** _____ **Completed by:** _____					
Issue—Mark Each as Yes; No; n/a	MR No.	MR No.	MR No.	MR No.	MR No.
Observation measure (actual number of behaviors observed/total number behaviors possible)					
18. The number of times hand hygiene was done/number of times hand hygiene should have been done (before and after patient care, staff breaks, eating, etc.).	/	/	/	/	/
19. Ask the nurse whether patient transporters are initiating the "ticket to ride."					
20. Refrigerator logs are being completed to document temperature checks.					
21. Code carts are being checked and documented daily.					
MR, medical record.					

types of charts can easily be constructed using standard computer programs. The type of chart needed will depend on the measures and the information needing analysis.

One of the most basic charts designed to identify trends in the variables is a run chart. Run charts are line graphs that display data over time and can show whether there has been a change in the performance after an intervention is implemented. One process or several can be shown on the same chart if the data are being analyzed for comparisons in trends. This type of chart is shown in **FIGURE 12-4**. This line (or run) in the chart depicts the process variation. All processes have variation that is either part of the process itself (common cause variation) or due to external influences (special cause variation) (Geary & Clanton, 2011; Lighter, 2011; Missel & Thomas, 2015). Being able to recognize the special cause variation is important, especially when analyzing for effects from an intervention. Run charts typically have the time interval on the horizontal axis and the variable being measured on the vertical axis. The data are plotted over time, and variation is evaluated. Two special cause trends are runs and shifts. Runs mean there is a continual increase or decrease seen for six data points in a row, and shifts cause data points to all fall above or below the average or centerline. Runs and shifts need to be analyzed further in order to determine the cause of the variation.

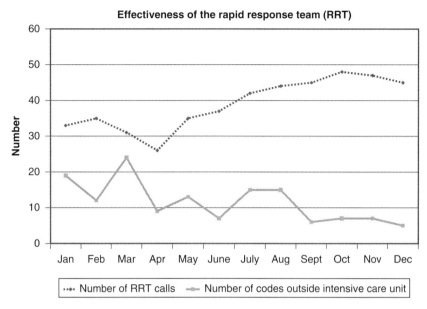

FIGURE 12-4 Run Chart Comparing Two Processes: Rapid Response Team Calls and Codes

Control charts are run charts that include the process parameters of mean and standard deviation calculated from the process data. These parameters make the centerline (mean) and the upper and lower control limits. The control limits are determined by adding or subtracting the standard deviation to or from the mean. Control limits can be set as one, two, or three standard deviations above and below the process mean depending on what is being measured and how much variance is acceptable. The more standard deviations used, the larger the control limits and the more variation is accepted before the process is said to need additional analysis. So if the control chart is trending serious patient issues (mortalities, infections, etc.), the control limits would best be set at one or two standard deviations so that only minimum occurrences would be tolerated. Both the run chart and control chart are useful tools to use when analyzing data over time to determine if a process is performing as designed or if a change has occurred—whether intentional, unintentional, positive, or negative. If data stay within the control limits, the process is stable. The process is unstable when data points are found to be outside of the control limits, and further investigation is needed to determine the special cause(s) of the variation. In the control chart example shown in **FIGURE 12-5**, there are 3 months when the number of patients leaving the emergency department before they were seen were outside the control limits. All three of these months should be further reviewed to determine any specific causes or common factors (Geary & Clanton, 2011).

Two types of bar charts that are useful for analyzing the frequency or pattern of the data over a time period are histograms and Pareto charts. A histogram, as shown in **FIGURE 12-6**, is used to determine if the process has a normal distribution. Data are said to be bell shaped or normally distributed when the most frequent data appear within the center of the graph, with equal data points appearing on either side (Geary & Clanton, 2011; Okes & Westcott, 2001; Wescott, 2013). An abnormal

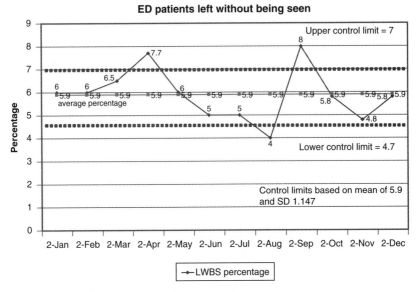

FIGURE 12-5 Control Chart with Mean, Standard Deviations

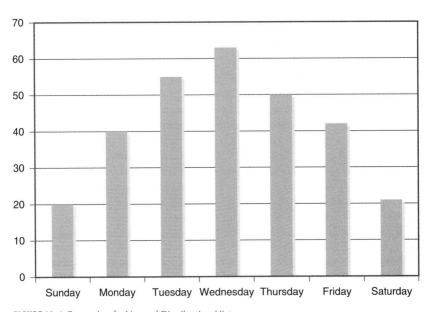

FIGURE 12-6 Example of a Normal Distribution Histogram

distribution or shape indicates that the process is not performing as designed and additional review is needed.

A Pareto chart is a bar chart that shows the frequency of measures. This type of graph is based upon the Pareto principle, which states that 80% of the process variation, or cause of a problem, is based on 20% of the variables (Geary & Clanton, 2011; Okes & Westcott, 2001; Wescott, 2013). The bars in the Pareto chart are ranked in

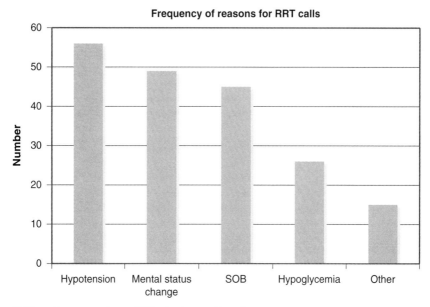

RRT, rapid response team; SOB, shortness of breath.

FIGURE 12-7 Pareto Chart Showing Most Frequent to Least Frequent Reason for RRT Calls

descending frequency with the variables listed on the horizontal axis and frequency on the vertical axis. In **FIGURE 12-7**, the most frequent cause identified for calling the rapid response team is patients having hypotension. Being able to make this analysis helps direct any additional information needed to identify any common factors contributing to these patients developing hypotension.

The last chart that is helpful in analyzing data is a scatter diagram. Scatter diagrams are useful in determining if there is a correlation between two variables. A positive correlation is indicated when there is an upward slope found among the data points. A negative correlation is seen when the pattern slopes downward, which occurs when one variable's increase correlates with the other variable's decrease. When there is not an identifiable pattern found, the scatter diagram is interpreted as showing there is no correlation between the two variables. A positive or negative correlation does not necessarily mean there is a direct cause-and-effect relationship between the two variables. There is also no way to determine the strength of the correlation from a scatter diagram. Additional measurement would be needed for that type of analysis. The first step involved in constructing a scatter diagram is to determine the variables and the type of relationship being investigated (cause/cause; cause/effect). Next, obtain paired data for the two variables and place the cause on the horizontal axis and the effect on the vertical axis. Finally, plot the data and check for any patterns. Patterns are interpreted as positive correlations, no correlations, or negative correlations, as shown in **FIGURE 12-8**. (Geary & Clanton, 2011)

It is important to have a data management plan to determine the measures needed to support and evaluate any project or new program. Many different hospital departments perform ongoing measurement to evaluate different processes and outcomes. Some of these measures are suitable to use to evaluate and analyze new

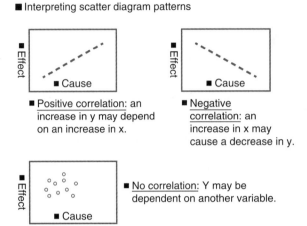

FIGURE 12-8 Different Correlations Found in Scatter Diagrams

aspects of care, but often additional data are needed to be able to do a true analysis of an issue. If additional measures are needed, then the most direct measurement of the concept should be considered. Also, there are always new questions raised when analyzing a project or program. Using the appropriate statistical process tools will contribute to a comprehensive analysis and guide decision-making (Geary & Clanton, 2011).

▶ Summary

- In this era of health reform where quantifying both cost and quality garner equal attention, it is incumbent on the profession to develop skills and confidence in measuring the impact of our work.
- For many, the prospect of selecting metrics instills fear given their importance in creating a powerful story to share with others about the contributions nurses make with their work. Recognizing the stature of nurses within healthcare delivery, *The Future of Nursing: Leading Change, Advancing Health* (2010) written by the Robert Wood Johnson Foundation and the Institute of Medicine identified, as a key message, the need to partner fully with members of the healthcare team and improve the information data infrastructure to support decision-making and policy making directed to improved health outcomes for the nation. Inherent in this is the ability to manage projects, establish evidence, and distinguish appropriate metrics and measurement for change outcomes.
- As healthcare delivery system is reformed, an essential lever will be measuring meaningful elements of our practice to improve outcomes. This will include a thoughtful data plan as well as appropriate metrics.
- Building from what has been learned about research and evidence-based practice implementation, the disciplines of project management and quality improvement serve as the guardrails for selection of meaningful metrics.

Reflection Questions

1. Consider the definitions of process and outcome indicators. Select an area of practice you believe a project could be developed for. What are some of the process metrics you might consider to demonstrate progress or improvements in care? What are some of the outcome measures you would consider?

2. You are having lunch with a colleague who works on a different unit. She has heard about a program that is being developed to serve the patient population you care for. She doesn't understand how the decisions were made about data that will be analyzed. How would you explain the decision-making process for selecting metrics?

3. Reflect on your current practice. Where would you go to get information about data available in your organization? Data in the electronic medical record? Administrative data? Claims data? Datasets or data warehouse? Who are the people (or roles and departments) to help you develop knowledge and understanding of the available data?

References

Agency for Healthcare Research and Quality (AHRQ) National Quality Measures Clearinghouse. (2014). *Uses of quality measures*. Retrieved from: http://www.qualitymeasures.ahrq.gov/tutorial/using.aspx

Andre, B., & Sjovold, E. (2017). What characterizes the work culture at a hospital unit that successfully implements change—a correlation study. *BMC Health Services Research, 17*(486). http://dx.doi.org/10.1186/s12913-017-2436-4

Bodenheimer, T., & Sinsky, C. (2014). From triple to quadruple aim: Care of the patient requires care of the provider. *Annals of Family Medicine, 12*(6), 573–576.

Brown, B., & Hough-Falk, L. (2014). Embarking on performance improvement. *Healthcare Financial Management, 68*(6), 98–103.

Brown, D., Aydin, C., & Donaldson, N. (2008). Quartile dashboards: Translating large data sets into performance improvement priorities. *Journal for Healthcare Quality, 30*(6), 18–30.

Centers for Medicare and Medicaid Services CMS. HCAHPS: Patients' Perspectives of care survey. Retrieved from at http://www.cms.gov/Medicare/Quality-Initiatives-Patient-Assessment-Instruments/HospitalQualityInits/HospitalHCAHPS.html

Datsenko, Y., & Schenk, J. (2013). Leading clinical projects. *Applied Clinical Trials Online, 22*(1), 22–28.

Geary, M., & Clanton, C. (2011). Developing metrics that support projects and programs. In J. Harris, L. Roussel, S. Walters, & C. Dearman, *Project planning and management: A guide for CNLs, DNPs, and nurse executives.* Sudbury, MA: Jones & Bartlett Learning.

Hadfield, D., Holmes, S., Kozlowski, S., Sperl, T., & Tapping, D. (2012). *The new lean healthcare pocket guide: Tools for the elimination of waste in hospitals, clinics, and other healthcare facilities. Chelsea,* MI: MCS Media, Inc.

Hall, H., & Roussel, L. (2014). *Evidence-based practice: An integrative approach to research, administration, and practice.* Burlington MA: Jones & Bartlett Learning.

Hoff, T., & Sutcliffe, K. (2006). Studying patient safety in health care organizations: Accentuate the qualitative. *The Joint Commission Journal on Quality and Patient Safety, 32*(1), 5–15.

Institute for Healthcare Improvement (IHI). (2015a). *How to improve.* Retrieved from http://www.ihi.org/resources/Pages/HowtoImprove/default.aspx

Institute for Healthcare Improvement (IHI). (2015b). *The IHI triple aim.* Retrieved from http://www.ihi.org/Engage/Initiatives/TripleAim/Pages/default.aspx

Institute of Medicine (IOM). (1999). *To err is human: Building a safer health system.* Washington, DC: National Academies Press.

Institute of Medicine (IOM). (2001). *Crossing the quality chasm: A new health system for the 21st century.* Washington, DC: National Academy Press.

Institute of Medicine (IOM). (2003). *Health professions education: A bridge to quality*. Washington, DC: National Academies Press.

Ko, C. Y. (2009, November/December). Measuring and improving surgical quality. *Patient Safety and Quality Healthcare*. Retrieved from https://www.psqh.com/analysis/measuring -and-improving-surgical-quality

Kurtzman, E., Dawson, E., & Johnson, J. (2008). The current state of nursing performance measurement, public reporting and value-based purchasing. *Policy, Politics & Nursing, 9*(3), 181–190.

Lam, M., & Robertson, D. (2012). Culture, tenure, and willingness to participate in continuous improvement projects in healthcare. *The Quality Management Journal, 19*(3), 7–15.

Lighter, D. E. (2011). *Advanced performance improvement in health care: Principles and methods*. Sudbury, MA: Jones & Bartlett Learning.

Malloch, K., & Porter-O'Grady, T. (2010). *Introduction to evidence-based practice in nursing and health care* (2nd ed.). Sudbury, MA: Jones and Bartlett Publishers.

Melnyk, B. M., & Fineout-Overholt, E. (2015). *Evidence-based practice in nursing & healthcare: A guide to best practice* (3rd ed.). Philadelphia, PA: Wolters Kluwer.

Missel, A., & Thomas, P. (2015). Developing metrics that support projects and programs. In J. Harris, L. Roussel, C. Dearman, & P. Thomas, *Project planning and management: A guide for nurses and interprofessional teams* (2nd ed.). Burlington, MA: Jones & Bartlett Learning.

National Quality Forum. (2010). *Safe practices for better healthcare—2010 update*. Retrieved from http://www.qualityforum.org/Publications/2010/04/Safe_Practices_for_Better_Healthcare_–_2010 _Update.aspx

Nelson, E., Batalden, P., & Godfrey, M. (2007). *Quality by design: A clinical microsystems approach*. San Francisco, CA: Jossey-Bass.

Okes, D., & Westcott, R. (2001). *The certified quality manager handbook*. Milwaukee, WI: American Society for Quality Press Publications.

Polit, D., & Beck, C. (2004). *Nursing research: Principles and methods* (7th ed.). Philadelphia, PA: Lippincott Williams & Wilkins.

Press Ganey. (2014, June 10). Press Ganey acquires national database of nursing quality indicators (NDNQI®). *PR Newswire*. Retrieved from https://www.prnewswire.com/news-releases/press -ganey-acquires-national-database-of-nursing-quality-indicators-ndnqi-262538811.html

Press Ganey. (2017). *Nursing quality: Improve care quality, prevent adverse events with deep nursing quality insights*. Retrieved from http://www.pressganey.com/solutions/clinical-quality/nursing-quality

Radnor, Z., Holweg, M., & Waring, J. (2012). Lean in healthcare: The unfilled promise? *Social Science & Medicine, 74*, 364–371.

Robert Wood Johnson Foundation & The Institute of Medicine. (2010). *The future of nursing: Leading change, advancing health*. Retrieved from http://www.nationalacademies.org/hmd/Reports/2010 /The-Future-of-Nursing-Leading-Change-Advancing-Health.aspx

Schein, E. (2004). *Organizational culture and leadership* (3rd ed.). San Francisco, CA: Jossey-Bass.

Shank, G. (2006). *Qualitative research* (2nd ed.). Upper Saddle River, NJ: Pearson.

Sheppy, B., Zuliani, J., & McIntosh, B. (2012). Science or art: Risk and project management in healthcare. *British Journal of Healthcare Management, 18*(11), 586–590.

Shirley, D. (2011). *Project management for healthcare*. Boca Raton, FL: CRC Press.

The Joint Commission. (2017). *Hospital standards CAMH*. Retrieved from https://www.jointcommission .org/standards_information/hap_requirements.aspx

Wescott, R. (2013). *The certified manager of quality: Organizational excellence handbook* (4th ed.). Milwaukee, WI: American Society for Quality Press Publications.

Williams, T., & Geary, M. (1997). *Improving nursing performance*. Chicago, IL: Precept Press.

CHAPTER 13

Measuring the Value of Projects Within Organizations, Healthcare Systems, and Globally

Patricia L. Thomas
Michael Bleich

CHAPTER OBJECTIVES

1. Define value in project management.
2. Explore principles of project evaluation.
3. Identify team attributes, engaging experts, and project oversight responsibilities.
4. Describe communication requirements and dissemination strategies.

KEY TERMS

Communication
Dissemination
Evaluation plan

Evidence
Information management
Value

ROLES

Communicator	Integrator
Decision-maker	Leader
Influencer	Risk anticipator
Information manager	

PROFESSIONAL VALUES

Altruism	Social justice
Integrity	

CORE COMPETENCIES

Assessment	Evaluation
Coordination	Interpersonal influence
Critical thinking/appreciative inquiry	Leadership
Data analysis	Measurement
Data management	Risk reduction
Design	Systems thinking
Emotional intelligence	

▶ Introduction

When an organization undertakes a project, a major driver in decision-making is intention to align the work with the organization's mission and vision. Strategic alignment with the mission leverages priority for constrained resources to be assigned to the proposed project. Allocating resources for a project typically requires shifting existing resources away from one project or program for use in the proposed project. This simple frame belies the essence of this chapter—that **value** must be attained and measured to ensure that the allocation of resources did, in fact, advance the organization's mission and vision and that the investment of resources into the project yielded value to stakeholders.

Measuring value is difficult, both conceptually and practically. In recent years, significant efforts to establish consistent data definitions for reporting and transparency purposes have emerged that highlight key attributes of cost-effective, high-quality, low-cost care. Notably, the Institute for Healthcare Improvement's Triple Aim, to provide quality care to populations served that is efficient, effective, and low cost, serves as a framework and driver for care improvement. The Centers for Medicare and Medicaid Services (CMS) hospital, home care, and skilled nursing facility compare websites provide information on location-specific quality indicators and core measure benchmarks that define cost and quality parameters achieved in organizations. The Hospital Quality Alliance, accreditors, regulators, and third-party payors have created and generated evidence and reporting mechanisms to influence organizational priorities for resource allocation to promote efforts that demonstrate value-added care delivery.

In 2012, CMS introduced value-based purchasing, a program that provides incentive payments for the quality of care in hospitals, hospitals, home health, and skilled nursing facilities. Centered on the Triple Aim, value-based programs move away from the quantity of care provided (volume) to the quality of care. Incentives also align to readmission rates and hospital-acquired conditions (CMS, 2017).

▶ How Value Is Defined in Health Care

In recent years, U.S. healthcare spending, representing nearly 18% of the gross domestic product (GDP) or nearly $3 trillion, has stabilized compared to predicted long-term spending trends; however, sustainability of the system remains a concern. The Institute of Medicine stated, "the only sensible way to restrain costs is to enhance the value of the system, thus extracting more benefit from the dollars spent" (IOM, 2013, p. xi). With this context, improving productivity, efficiency, effectiveness, and coordination of care are foci for value-added processes, projects, and programs. While much has been written about quality improvement, project design, and measurement as vehicles to hardwire evidence-based practices in care delivery, variation in practice, care delivery, and outcomes remains. Now, coequal partner concepts, cost, and quality are cornerstones in healthcare debates, policy making, and care delivery decisions where in the past, quality reigned as the principal goal. Irrespective of the project or program, measurement of financial impacts is a necessity and inclusion and transparency related to cost are key to the credibility of the team, project sponsor, and project manager.

▶ Measurement

To generate value, measurement of information is needed, usually drawn from databases but often collected specifically for a project, based on anticipated and desired outcomes. The information collected must be informative, meaning that a predesigned plan for its use has been determined. If it informs, then it must also be relevant to the project and sensitive so that it measures real differences in the project's anticipated impact. Further, information must be unbiased and comprehensive to capture the scope and magnitude of the project, such that the integrity of the project's impact is real. Measuring the impact of a project also requires timely information. Additionally, how that information is stored and maintained must be considered so that impact can be measured throughout the project's duration and in sustainability. In project management, information must be performance targeted to the goals and objectives of the project, collected in a uniform manner, and, importantly, cost-effective and possible to obtain. These attributes, as per Austin (1979), have been a foundation for project management and quality improvement changes over time.

The next challenge is how to capture value. While the cost or expense of a service can define value, the healthcare industry has, at its foundation, people and the experiences they have through interacting with care providers. The perceptions of care held by all stakeholders, patients, family members, employees, and care-providing professional disciplines, and the organization's governing board, are guided by their unique and shared interests. Value is expressed by first knowing what the stakeholders' interests are. In the case of a project that influences organizational efficiencies, this may be measured in time saved, simplifying a complex task, replacing a way of working that is distasteful with one that is opposite, supplanting one method for another, and the like. There may be dimensions of cost-effectiveness, job autonomy, and other factors. The project manager must be clear about the stakeholders' needs and wants to form baseline for comparison of outcomes. Similarly, if the project impacts patient care, then the patient's perceptions must be considered. Will the project create ease of access to care? Or will it provide for symptom management, influence quality of life, diminish pain or discomfort, or reduce the advancement of disease to a higher stage of chronicity? The project leader must be clear about the aim of the project and establish this from a value perspective. As stated earlier, measuring value is complex and requires considerable forethought and design (Fitzgerald, 2004; Koomans & Hilders, 2017). This is an often-missed step in healthcare project improvement initiatives.

If it is not already apparent, the project manager will play multiple roles in the measurement of project value. Measuring value and impact of any project must be considered during design and before the onset of the project activities. The project manager must understand the genesis of the project, especially when a project is delegated as an opportunity for visibility and growth of the project manager. What were the organizational dynamics that led to the project? What are the strategic and operational impacts desired from the project? Who are the affected stakeholders? What, in the creation of change, is going to be lost and gained as a result of the project? The role of leadership comes into play by venturing into the unknown. The role of manager is executed by guiding the project through a defined process. But additional roles germane to this chapter are also relevant: The project manager must be strategic and must function as a planner, the **communicator** (which includes being a sleuth in order to understand people, processes, and structures that influence the project), a data analyst, and even a database administrator. Value, then, based on stakeholder expectations, may be expressed in terms of time saved, cost, convenience, access, simplicity of use, and more.

▶ Project Evaluation

A common and accepted definition of project evaluation is, "The systematic collection of information about the activities, characteristics, and outcomes of program, services, policy, or processes, in order to make judgments about the program/ process, improve effectiveness, and/or inform decisions about future development." (Bowen, 2012, p. 6). With this context, program evaluation informs management decisions where evaluation research generates knowledge that may be applicable to other settings. Value and valuing are central to evaluation. Scriven (1991) defined evaluation as "the process of determining the merit, worth, or value of something, or the product of that process" (p. 139), emphasizing that descriptive data are not evaluation. Evaluation is often used to improve and demonstrate the merit of programs or activities (summative evaluation) or to improve or refine a program (formative evaluation). In the design or development of a program, developmental evaluation is used. Where knowledge is limited, evaluation may be used to generate new knowledge (Bowen, 2012).

▶ Steps in Program Evaluation

While activities of program evaluation are presented sequentially, it is often an iterative process that can be worked through different orders. Typically, a program evaluation includes:

1. Considering the evaluation purpose
2. Identifying stakeholders
3. Assessing evaluation expertise
4. Gathering relevant evidence
5. Building consensus (Bowen, 2012)

▶ Aligning Metrics with Project Aims

Projects vary in terms of the magnitude and scope of the change, the stakeholders involved, and the degree of linearity or complexity associated with the approach taken to manage the project. **TABLE 13-1** provides a useful framework for examining a project's level of complexity (Berger, 2005).

An example of a simple project might be the introduction of a product that is available at the point of care to encourage hand hygiene. The aim of the project has a defined location (bedside), a defined targeted audience (bedside caregivers), and a targeted aim (nosocomial infection reduction or prevention). As simple as this might seem, the project leader must consider what to measure. Should we measure hand-washing compliance using the product? Should we measure changes in nosocomial infection rates? Will we measure the impact of the product in real time or retrospectively? Is there an existing database from which to draw information? Does one need to be created? Will we sample for outcomes or include the entire population? When is the best time to collect the data to represent the results with integrity and to reduce risk? Who will collect the data, and how will data collection be coordinated? From this example, there are many clues to indicate that the complexities of measuring value are endless.

▶ Case Study Application

A project manager has been appointed based on a community desire to be more heart healthy. The hospital responded favorably to this community request, which emanated from several organizations, including the YMCA, the statewide affiliate of the American Heart Association, and civic leaders whose concern was a healthy workforce. A cardiovascular nurse leader was selected by the hospital CEO to lead the hospital's efforts to make a huge impact on cardiovascular health. The project aims included assuring that exercise was available to all age groups year-round, having one or more citizens trained in CPR reside on every city block, and placing a defibrillator device in all public buildings with an occupancy of 75 or more people. Note that, fortunately, the project aims were all measurable, which is not always the case.

The nurse leader charged with this project had a number of complex design challenges to think through, beginning with a willing spirit and strong personal values that the project was a good thing. Using **TABLE 13-1** as a reference, the nurse determined that

TABLE 13-1 Project Characteristics as a Precursor to Metric Selection

Simple Project	Mid-Range Project	Complex Project
Stakeholders are limited to a select few, often with readily aligned values and needs.	Stakeholders are modest in number and cross boundaries within an organizational setting where values and needs are similar.	Stakeholders are large in number or are of varying disciplines with often disparate values and needs.
The project is primarily linear with clearly defined outcomes targeted at individuals and groups.	The project is both linear and nonlinear in that the outcomes extend to influence behaviors that are less defined and that focus at the group level of attainment.	The project is primarily nonlinear with less defined structure, and the outcomes cannot be clearly defined and are aimed at social change.
The project manager retains the ability to oversee and control each aspect of project activities.	The project manager works with a team to oversee and provide general direction while the project unfolds and morphs to meet unanticipated needs.	The project manager does not exist in one individual but rather extends to intersecting groups, all of whom share a common aim, and multiple strategies emerge to shape the direction of the project.
Metrics are simple to retrieve from existing data and can be readily observed or collected; feedback loops are easy to define and are often from a single source.	Metrics are retrieved from multiple data sources and may require development beyond what is available, with feedback loops required from multiple sources.	Metrics are retrieved from large databases and public opinion and must capture the multiple interests within divergent populations and stakeholders.
Metrics are focused on project completion and simple outcomes.	Metrics are focused on organizational impact and more complex outcomes, beyond project completion to project impact.	Metrics are focused on social change with complex social outcomes.
The value to measure is tied to a few defined concepts within a narrow range.	The value to measure is tied to multiple concepts within a broad organizational range.	The value to measure is tied to social concepts that cross organizational boundaries.

there were components of the project that could be subdivided and that crossed over all project levels from simple to complex. The leader recognized that the project had dimensions that addressed social justice and that there was an altruistic component to it. **Evidence** about cardiovascular disease supported the project and could be used for ideas about measuring the project's impact. Evidence that did not already exist also needed to be gathered. The following questions needed to be answered: How many establishments exist that accommodate 75 or more people? How many have automatic external defibrillators? Further, how many city blocks exist, and where do the city limits end? Does the charter really mean city blocks, or should suburbs be included? What are the ramifications if they are not included? What is the anticipated risk of limiting the project to the city? How does one define *exercise*? What are socially acceptable norms relating to exercise given weather conditions and public safety issues? How will the communities of interest value and accept the risk associated with exercise or the lack thereof?

Only when these and similar questions were answered could an effective metric design and **information management** plan emerge. Systems thinking was needed by the nurse leader to understand the interrelated components of the project and to recognize which parts of the project had linear, systematic, and predictable components to them versus other aspects of the project that targeted larger social and policy issues. In a brainstorming session around metrics, the following suggestions emerged:

- We could collect data on satisfaction with CPR training.
- We could count the number of individuals who exercise on a regular basis.
- We could look at the number of heart-related procedures that are performed at the local hospital and see if those go down.
- We could look at claims databases to check for cardiac risk factors.
- We could mandate that vending machines have their food choices altered to include healthy alternatives and count the changes.
- We could count the number of people who attend a health fair and have their blood pressure taken.
- We could restrict public smoking because of its link to heart disease and monitor heart disease occurrences.
- We could count the number of new exercise programs that are held in public places, including long-term-care facilities.

If you were going to use this list, how useful would it be to you? Which data are tied to simple, mid-range, and complex social change? How accessible is the information suggested? Is it performance targeted? Are they new or existing data? How do the data tie to the project objectives set forth? How do the metrics suggested integrate with the project? What would you change?

▶ Principles of Project Evaluation Methods

Project evaluation is an effort to measure the impact of project-based change. The value proposition to be measured is derived from the stakeholders themselves, which often are diverse. One stakeholder (e.g., a shareholder) may have a singular interest in profit. Another stakeholder (e.g., a patient) may have an interest in access, cost, and quality. Regulators may want adherence to a defined set of standards. Many projects evolve from quality improvement initiatives, where metrics are a close "cousin" to project management metrics. In fact, the principles of developing metrics for quality improvement serve as a substantive guide for project evaluation (Berger, 2005; Bowen, 2012; Lloyd, 2004).

In order to adequately meet the needs of the stakeholders, the project manager (note that this is not a formal title but rather a temporary job assignment, such as in the case study) bears responsibility for measuring the impact of project objectives or aims. These objectives should be readily aligned with the organization's mission and purpose if the level of change is targeted within an institutional setting. But some projects extend to multiple settings and are therefore more complex for determining a single value proposition. Insurance companies may have a desire to provide different health education, for instance, than what is desired by a provider–patient relationship. These differences must be accounted for in complex changes.

Some researchers describe project evaluation methods as being closely aligned with the field of program evaluation. As defined by Fink (1993), program evaluation is a diligent investigation of a program's characteristics and merits. Its purpose is to provide information on the effectiveness of projects so as to optimize the outcomes, efficiency, and quality of health care. Evaluations can analyze a program's structure, activities, and organization and examine its political and social environment. They can also appraise the achievements of a project's goals and objectives and the extent of its impact and costs.

Fink (1993) differentiated project and program evaluation from other types of research in that its major task is to judge a program's merits. She defined a meritorious program/project as one that has "worthy goals, achieves its standards of effectiveness, provides benefits to its participants, fully informs its participants of potential risks of participation, and does no harm" (1993, p. 2). Developing value metrics in an organizational context, then, can relate to measuring program objectives and activities, program outcomes, and program impact.

The methods used to capture data include both quantitative and qualitative strategies. As used here, quantitative methods include approaches that measure impact through mechanisms such as data retrieval from existing administrative and national databases; economic cost-effectiveness determination; surveys measuring perceptions; and targeted research instruments that measure patient, family, and societal outcomes that align with the project objectives and aims. Examples of quantitative data include selecting metrics from the following:

- Clinical/epidemiologic databases, such as those contained in disease registries or through epidemiologic surveys (Johantgen, 2005)
- Administrative claims data at the organization or state level (Johantgen, 2005)
- Sociodemographic data, such as that available through census reports and state-level vital statistics records
- Patient satisfaction data, such as that available through proprietary databases at the institutional level (Hayes, 2008)
- National Data on Nursing Quality Indicators (NDNQI) data, applied at the institutional level (Montalvo, 2007; Trossman, 2006)
- Marketing data that specify lifestyle and other useful population practices

Similarly, qualitative data provide rich context for project impact. These data are available through the following:

- Focus groups with project-oriented aims
- Appreciative inquiry/storytelling methods aligned with stakeholder groups (Whitney & Trosten-Bloom, 2003)
- Internet and social networking approaches to capture context

▶ Information Dissemination: Roles and Responsibilities for Communication

The project manager has the ultimate responsibility to ensure that the impact of project implementation is reflected in useful ways to stakeholder groups. As early data are collected, the **dissemination** of information is critical to the stabilization of the project. Those engaged in the change need and want feedback on how the project is progressing. While the full impact of change may be unknown in the early stages of data collection, it does provide motivation toward meeting project aims and objectives. Chapter 14 gives greater detail on the dissemination process.

Face-to-face **communication** is helpful, but when it comes to data presentation, it simply is not enough. The accountable project manager displays data using charts, survey tools, graphs, and other means to fully reflect the impact of the project during its implementation and at the conclusion of the intervention and continues to monitor postintervention effectiveness and restabilization. Today, electronic support of data presentation and analysis underscores the need to be transparent in all facets of program accountability.

Rarely do projects turn out exactly as planned. If the right metrics are selected, namely, those that show sensitivity to the project aims and objectives, and if the data are reliably collected and displayed, then variation will occur from the plan. This does not mean failure of the project but, rather, presents an opportunity for the project leader and stakeholder groups to "torture the data," as John Ruskin was quoted as saying, such that meaning emerges from the data (Ruskin, 2010). In other words, data themselves do not signify the success or failure of a project. Only collective meaning and an eye toward improvement derive a project's success. Too often, project managers feel the obligation to measure that which appears to denote success rather than capture what is successful—or not—about a project.

The presentation of feedback through quantitative and qualitative data presents the opportunity for the project leader to anticipate risk, integrate findings with lived reality, communicate a sense of purpose to the stakeholders, and design plans for improving the project past its due date and into the fabric of the work of the organization.

Especially in the case of projects that lead to system change, the use of statistical process control charts helps to determine the impact of the change and resets the new and improved standard, such that variation can be identified as that which is created by the system change itself (known as common cause variation) or as a major aberrancy that rests outside of the system change (special cause variation) (Deming, 1986). These techniques, used in quality improvement, are critical to help determine whether a changed system is performing in a desirable manner and quickly draw attention to special causes that are not related to the change itself. Although outside of the scope of this chapter, statistical process control tools should be within the realm of project managers to aid in decision-making and direction setting (Carey & Lloyd, 2001).

Lastly, it is important to portray the effects of change to stakeholder groups. A final report, a summary email, a closure event to mark achievements, or the presence of run charts with notes attached to denote accomplishments are all mechanisms that can be employed to tell the story of the value that the project brought to the organization, its stakeholders, and others who evaluate the organization, such as external regulators, public constituency groups, and the like. Today, nurse leaders are not present often enough in the boardroom to discuss change, but a well-educated project leader, with the right tools for communication and data presentation, should be present at the venue to advance patient care and to inform others of the contributions of nursing and other healthcare professionals.

▶ Tools of the Trade

In project management, inexpensive statistical process control software is readily available. Some basic procedures can be performed with an Excel spreadsheet. When these tools are used, the process changes that have occurred can be monitored for common cause and special cause variation, as described previously. The control chart that emanates from statistical process control powerfully documents change and variability (Kelley, 1999).

Similarly, graphic presentation of data is useful, particularly when it can be modeled in a dashboard style of presentation. A dashboard presentation compares and contrasts metrics into a single document, such that patient outcomes, staff performance, economic data, and risk data, for example, can be studied as a set, aiding decision-making by displaying that one variable (e.g., cost savings) is not working against other variables (e.g., patient satisfaction). This is another important tool for decision-making and evaluation (Nelson, 1995).

▶ Summary

- Value is about knowing the specific stakeholder wants and needs related to the project. These can vary widely but often include access to service, cost-effective delivery of service, and satisfaction with the project's outcomes.
- Measuring value depends on the art and science of selecting metrics. Metrics must be informative, relevant, unbiased and comprehensive, action oriented, performance targeted, and cost-effective.
- Projects vary in complexity, and the metrics will vary accordingly.
- Metrics can include both quantitative and qualitative data; the former provides information about specific points of achievement, whereas the latter provides context. They are complementary.
- Project leaders are accountable for a fair and honest representation of the project and should be prepared to reveal progress toward the aims, as well as unanticipated outcomes, both positive and negative.
- Project leaders should use decision science tools, such as those associated with statistical process control and dashboard mapping, to represent their work and to adapt projects as needed.
- Data should support the project from before the onset of the project through to project stabilization, until the work is sustained as part of the way work is done.

Reflection Questions

1. What is the importance of defining a clear end-point vision prior to implementing a project? What role should stakeholders play in articulating this vision?
2. What role does standards setting play in selecting metrics? Does the role of Donabedian's (2003) structure → process → outcome model play have any relevance in choosing metrics?

3. How do the research principles of data validity and reliability tie into data collection in project management? Do data that do not have confirmed validity and reliability play any role in evaluation?
4. How does one determine the cost of data collection and management compared to its relative value in project evaluation?

Learning Activities

1. Take an existing project and determine whether or not clear outcomes for the project were stated early on in the project. Examine who the stakeholders were/should have been to establish these outcomes. Did a data collection plan exist that would measure the impact of the project?
2. Develop measurable and obtainable metrics for a project. Include with these metrics an operational definition to focus on what the metric measures and how it ties to the project. Develop a sampling plan for data collection, including whether the data will be collected in real time or on a retrospective basis. Determine who will collect and display the data and whether it comes from an existing database or must be collected as new data. Prepare a plan for using the data at various phases during and after the project. Anticipate how the data will affect decision-making, and provide feedback to stakeholders.
3. Generate a project **evaluation plan** based on a proposed project. What information was readily available to support evaluation? What was missing? Was value considered as part of the overall data management plan, and were specific metrics identified related to value?

References

Austin, C. (1979). *Information systems for hospital administration*. Ann Arbor, MI: Health Administration Press.

Berger, S. (2005). *The power of clinical and financial metrics: Achieving success in your hospital*. Chicago, IL: Health Administration Press.

Bowen, S. (2012). A guide to evaluation in health research. *Canadian Institutes of Health Research*. Retrieved from http://www.cihr-irsc.gc.ca/e/45336.html

Carey, R. G., & Lloyd, R. C. (2001). *Measuring quality improvement in healthcare: A guide to statistical process control applications*. Milwaukee, WI: ASQ Quality Press.

Centers for Medicare and Medicaid Services (CMS). (2017). *What are the value-based programs?* Retrieved from https://www.cms.gov/Medicare/Quality-Initiatives-Patient-Assessment-Instruments/Value-Based-Programs/Value-Based-Programs.html

Deming, W. E. (1986). *Out of the crisis*. Cambridge, MA: MIT Press.

Donabedian, A. (2003). *An introduction to quality assurance in health care*. New York, NY: Oxford University Press; 2003.

Fink, A. (1993). *Evaluation fundamentals: Guiding health programs, research, and policy*. Newbury Park, CA: Sage.

Fitzgerald, M. (2004, July 15). Don't stop thinking about the value. *CIO Magazine, 17*(19), 66.

Hayes, B. E. (2008). *Measuring customer satisfaction: Survey design, use, and statistical analysis methods* (3rd ed.). Milwaukee, WI: ASQ Quality Press.

Institute of Medicine (IOM). (2013). *Variation in health care spending: Target decision making, not geography*. Washington, DC: The National Academies Press.

Johantgen, M. (2005). Uses of existing administrative and national databases. In C. Waltz, O. L. Strickland, & E. R. Lenz (Eds.), *Measurement in nursing and health research* (pp. 326–338). New York, NY: Springer.

Kelley, D. L. (1999). *How to use control charts for healthcare.* Milwaukee, WI: ASQ Quality Press.

Koomans, M., & Hilders, C. (2017). Design-driven leadership for value innovation in healthcare. *Design Management Journal, 11*(1), 43–57.

Lloyd, R. (2004). *Quality health care: A guide to developing and using indicators.* Sudbury, MA: Jones and Bartlett Publishers.

Montalvo, I. (2007, September 30). The national database of nursing quality indicators (NDNQI). *The Online Journal of Issues in Nursing, 12*(3), Manuscript 2. https://doi.org/10.3912/OJIN .Vol12No03Man02

Nelson, E. (1995). Report cards or instrument panels: Who needs what? *Journal of Quality Improvement, 21*(4), 155–166.

Ruskin, J. (2010). *The complete works of John Ruskin: Stones of Venice, Volume III.* New York, NY: National Library Association.

Scriven, M. (1991). *Evaluation thesaurus* (4th ed.). Thousand Oaks, CA: Sage.

Trossman, S. (2006). Show us the data! NDNQI helps nurses link their care to quality. *The American Nurse, 38*(6), 1, 6.

Whitney, D., & Trosten-Bloom, A. (2003). *The power of appreciative inquiry: A practical guide to positive change.* San Francisco, CA: Berrett-Koehler Publishers.

CHAPTER 14

Disseminating Results of Meaningful Projects and Their Management

Catherine Dearman
Lolita Chappel-Aiken

PROFESSIONAL VALUES

Professionalism

CORE COMPETENCIES

Communication   Professionalism
Leadership

▶ Introduction

Dissemination of the results of projects and creative work promotes the exchange of information and extends the impact. It is essential to sustaining the innovation and to spreading the outcomes into various outlets. Dissemination of designs, processes, and outcomes allows others to truly understand the project and to determine how a similar project might work in their system. Without dissemination, potential consumers within and outside the primary organization will not be sufficiently aware of the project, which may impact use and overall outcomes.

Some projects naturally lend themselves to replicability within the system by the same team or similar teams. Replication of projects can, and arguably should, occur in other aspects of the primary agency or in other agencies or systems. Replicating a project can yield distinct positive results and serve to integrate the findings, resulting in improved sustainability and leading to quality improvement. Sustainability and replicability are inextricably linked to projects and the teams that produce them. Dissemination is not simply to promote replication of the project itself, rather, dissemination provides a sample or a plan as to how any innovation can be completed.

Dissemination can take many forms and to some extent depends on the venue in which the project took place. Nurse educators and those in the academic setting typically focus on the **publication** of articles in journals or the production of papers or **posters** for verbal presentation. Clinicians and nurse executives, in contrast, may seek to share their work at a more local or practice-based level. Many healthcare facilities working toward Magnet status must not only demonstrate that they have participated in quality improvement projects but also show that the processes and results of those projects have been disseminated and sustained throughout the system. Larger healthcare systems use projects and other creative, innovative works to advance team members on a career ladder. Dissemination is an integral part of all of those processes.

The true impact of a practice project or innovation is not always limited to one or more healthcare systems or even one form of dissemination. Some innovations are best shared through social media, on blogs, and even in "lay" literature such as women's or men's magazines.

This chapter addresses the dissemination of processes and outcomes through multiple venues and provides real-world information on preparing and delivering data to various groups and in a myriad of settings. The focus is on structuring the dissemination and methods of ascertaining submission requirements as well as on designing the actual dissemination itself. Dissemination is positively impacted when each person has and deliberately uses skills to enhance the delivery of the project outcomes. Use of a systems approach and appreciative inquiry methods provides an opportunity to capitalize on the skills and talents of the various team members who collectively produced and are disseminating the work.

▶ Professional Presentations

Most formal and many informal **presentations** involve the use of audio, audiovisual, or supportive technology, such as Microsoft's PowerPoint program, flip charts, story boards, video, and posters. The literature is replete with models or strategies to structure such presentations. Acronyms provide an easy method to remember the components the speaker needs to address in preparing a presentation. APPLE, which stands for audience, presentation, purpose, language, and evidence, provides a simple structure that is amenable to any presentation, whether one will address a group of students or peers or an international gathering of experts.

Audience

Consideration of the audience is critical to an effective presentation. Structuring a presentation that effectively represents the project and is predicated on the type of audience enhances the potential for a positive experience for each individual or group involved. Effective presentations reach out to and engage the audience as active participants in the experience.

The audience aspect of the APPLE model can represent the intended audience or the actual one. The intended audience is the group you are intending to reach, while the actual audience is the individuals who are exposed to the presentation. In any given venue, one may prepare a presentation for a group of like-minded individuals—but the attendees may not share the same view and, therefore, may respond in unexpected ways to the presentation. The presenter needs to be prepared to address the audience (intended or actual) effectively and manage the interaction in order to have a successful presentation.

Presentation

The presentation itself can be oral or written and may or may not include visual aids. Most presentations are planned, but some may take the form of spontaneous, off-the-cuff sharing of data. For example, a faculty member may be walking across campus when he or she is approached by a student or group of students who pose a question. The resulting dialogue could be termed a presentation of data, although little about it would be considered formal.

Personal preference and presentation style as well as the venue itself will guide whether the presentation is formal or informal. A research conference venue would naturally require statistical methods and data outcomes to be presented in a rather formal style. A conference designed to showcase teaching strategies or unit-specific interventions would highlight various teaching strategies and engender dialogue.

Most presentations include a question-and-answer session allowing the audience to fully engage with the content and the presenter. Successful interactions in these question-and-answer sessions can extend and expand the impact of the presentation. As one prepares to present, one should consider potential questions that may be raised by the audience and prepare to respond to them.

In many cases, an abstract of the presentation is provided to the audience, but in some cases, a full paper is required along with a verbal presentation. The abstract or paper is then included in a "proceedings" document for the conference. Proceedings documents count as publications, doubling the benefit to the presenter.

Poster presentations provide a more one-on-one opportunity to share the outcomes of the project with the audience. Poster presenters are asked to "man" their posters during breaks or exhibition times to allow the conference attendees to engage with the person or team who conducted the project and ask questions. A poster template is provided later in this chapter to guide content and placement.

Purpose

The purpose of the presentation has two primary aspects: explicit and implicit. The explicit purpose is the stated reason for the presentation; the implicit purpose is what the presenter ultimately hopes to accomplish. For example, one may express a primary purpose of a presentation as being to share the processes and outcomes of the project or innovation. The implicit purpose may be to further the presenter's career through sharing his or her scholarly work. The presenter's implicit purpose will, to some extent, shape the presentation and can make or break the outcome when combined with consideration of the audience and the presentation style.

The purpose of the presentation guides the development of the actual information to be presented and, combined with personal preference in style, will drive the manner in which the information is presented. For example, a researcher may wish to share his or her work very formally, fully describing the internal processes as well as the outcomes. Sharing the outcomes of a project in a less formal style may actually serve the overall purpose of the presentation by encouraging the audience to interact with the information and the presenter.

Language

The language component refers to the overall tone of the presentation including diction and formality, voice and tense, objectivity versus self-reference, and scientific/professional versus lay terminology or street language. The evidence or the information being conveyed can impact the language used in the presentation. The audience must be considered as well; the astute presenter watches audience reactions and adjusts the presentation accordingly. The language may be supported by data, facts, opinions, direct observations, references to the work of others, and hearsay, among other forms. Language and tone flexibility can significantly enhance the presentation, much the same as body language can impact a one-on-one interaction.

The presenter is responsible for tailoring the language to the audience and the venue. Failure to do so can negatively impact the entirety of the presentation. For example, if one prepares for a small, intimate gathering and encounters a large, boisterous audience, the language and style of presentation may need to be adjusted.

Engagement

Engaging the audience can entail maintaining eye contact, projecting a positive facial expression, and asking questions and eliciting responses, either verbal or nonverbal. Other methods of engaging the audience include ensuring that objectives match content, ensuring that the abstract or description provided to a potential audience is congruent with the actual presentation, and maintaining a less formal style. Engagement, like beauty, can frequently be in the eye of the beholder. Some people adopt a minimalistic personal style; others are effusive and ebullient. One's personal style may affect engagement in presentations offered in a different tone.

Remembering APPLE will facilitate the speaker being able to structure an effective presentation. Other considerations for podium presentations include honoring time constraints imposed by the conference to facilitate smooth operation. Extending over time impacts both audiences and other speakers.

Presentations may also occur as a group event or a panel discussion. In those cases, the time frame is for the entire group, not for each individual speaker. Participating as a part of a group or a panel typically means a far more restrictive environment, resulting in less opportunity for individual members of the group to tailor their personal presentations.

Visual and/or auditory aids are typically included along with the oral components of the presentation. Many speakers embed short videos or short computer interactions that make their point effectively and efficiently. If including these adjunctive methods, the speaker must be aware of the software and hardware interfaces available at the conference. Embedding a critical auditory or visual aid that is not effective in the venue can have a significant negative impact on the presentation. Presenters must always be aware that equipment may fail, be incompatible with the venue, be cumbersome, or be lost in transit; it is therefore critical to have a backup.

Additionally, entering the room allocated to the presentation in advance can lead to effective changes. For example, the size of the room typically reflects the number of anticipated attendees, which may impact handouts, visual aids, or presentation style. A large room may have "inappropriately" placed barriers such as posts which inhibit viewing. Finally, viewing a few slides from the presentation prior to beginning can assist the presenter with determining font size and color, the need for speakers to support audiovisual efforts, and a multitude of other considerations. In the case of presentations, it is generally better to be safe than sorry.

▶ Role of Appreciative Inquiry in Presentations

Appreciative inquiry (AI) is the coevolutionary search for the best in people, their organizations, and the relevant world around them. Appreciative inquiry gives life to a living system; presentations using AI provide an opportunity to share the hidden aspects of a system or a project that are not obvious to the audience. AI includes the art and practice of asking questions that strengthen a system's capacity to comprehend, anticipate, and heighten the positive potential of a project or innovation (Cooperrider & Whitney, 2010).

Traditionally, a project is not communicated until it is completed, and an innovation is not considered complete until outcomes are communicated. In AI, communication of outcomes occurs throughout the entire process of innovation, thereby creating transparency and an evidence-based culture (Marchionni & Richer, 2007). The approach to be used to communicate outcomes requires forethought, flexibility, willingness to capitalize on the differing presentation strengths of team members, and the ability to view the innovation process entirely.

The personal style of the presenter is critical to an effective presentation. The component of personal style addresses the unique strengths and characteristics that blend well with different people and situations at different times. Identifying and capitalizing on one's strengths and matching them to the characteristics of the intended audience increases the opportunity to make a truly successful presentation. When presenting early findings, matching one's personal style with the intended audience is especially critical. Early findings are more tenuous and can be ambiguous. Even skilled presenters can be challenged if the audience is not receptive to the data. Presentation of information about an innovation is considered successful if the information is remembered favorably and implemented or applied to new situations.

Personal style includes personal appearance, ease of interacting in different settings, vocal qualities (including volume, tone, pitch, and intonation), and personal power. Habitual and deliberate use of gestures, ease of making eye contact, ability to listen, ability to communicate interest and enthusiasm about the topic, and willingness to accept criticism can either add to or detract from a presentation. Being aware of one's personal style is essential to making effective presentations (Rutledge, Bajaj, & Mucciolo, 2007).

Ensuring the sustainability of an innovation requires understanding the various factors that influence its dissemination. Appreciative inquiry provides the context for disseminating results that directly contribute to sustaining innovations within systems by making the implicit connections more explicit. In other words, sustainability rests on presentations making essential hidden connections more obvious for all to see. The result is transparency for the team, the system, and the audience (Havens, Wood, & Leeman, 2006).

▶ Publications

Publications in academic circles are more valuable than other types of data sharing, such as posters, books, and book chapters. In this context, the word "publication" typically refers to an in-print or online paper that appears in a peer-reviewed journal. "Peer-reviewed" indicates a level of quality review that exceeds that performed in non-peer-reviewed or any other type of publication. Other terms indicating a peer review are "refereed" (as in "contested and emerging victorious") and "juried" (as in "from a jury of one's peers"). Academicians, especially those in competitive systems, consider only peer-reviewed publications when making tenure and promotion decisions. Although online publications are becoming more mainstream, print journals remain at the top of the academic pecking order.

Tappen (2011) provided the following advice for would-be authors seeking publication of their work in peer-reviewed journals: Endure criticism, maintain staying power, and tolerate revision. Seldom is one's paper accepted without revision. Other advice regarding peer-reviewed publications includes choosing the journal wisely (i.e., read the articles in the journal, look at the purpose and types of articles typically published, and tailor the submission to those elements). Additionally, authors should read and follow the journal's requirements; compile the literature review properly;

organize the paper appropriately with headings and other elements; proofread, proofread, proofread; format the manuscript correctly and double-check it; be willing and able to change the manuscript based on reviewers' comments; and refuse to concede defeat. Persistence and perseverance frequently win the day.

Books and book chapters are valuable learning and sharing tools, especially for those professionals early in their career or for health systems. Books and book chapters contain more of the surrounding details than can be shared in a poster or podium presentation and, therefore, are extremely useful for teaching others and for developing a strong writing style.

Posters are useful as mechanisms to share a lot of information quickly. A poster typically consists of a problem statement, findings, data elements, and outcomes. The poster presenter must consider how to provide these elements in a visually pleasing manner that is easy to read and understand (**FIGURE 14-1**). Poster sessions are frequently held during a conference at lunch or during breaks to allow larger exposure of presentations than can be accommodated with paper presentations. Poster presentations are far more informal and occur many times in a one-to-one fashion as interested audience members approach and read about the study. Handouts are especially helpful for poster presenters because they allow viewers to take the presentation with them.

Professional publications, presentations, books/chapters, and posters all share some commonalities in terms of preparation, such as tailoring the submission to the audience, being aware of the sponsor's requirements and ensuring that they are followed, and being tolerant of suggestions to improve. The final element is perhaps the most difficult to accept, especially when someone considers himself or herself to be the "expert" on the topic.

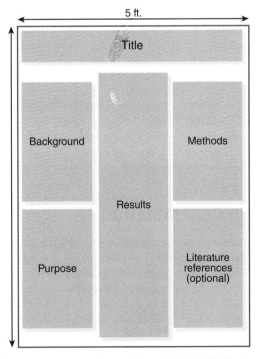

FIGURE 14-1 Sample Poster Format. Landscape Format is Desired for Display

▶ Other Types of Publications

Lay literature can be a valuable teaching tool for the general public. Academicians, however, would not presume to count a submission to a women's magazine or a newspaper as evidence of being deserving of tenure or promotion. That being said, publications that reach a wider population can be quite impactful, especially when the goal is to share "need-to-know" health information or to propose lifestyle changes. Many practitioners will find publication in lay journals to be as challenging as publication in peer-reviewed journals. Not only is the venue different, but the purpose and the manner in which the information is produced are vastly different. The same advice applies when submitting a manuscript to this type of publication: know the reputation and readership; follow directions; proofread; and take criticism well.

▶ Social and Informal Presentations

Social networking, such as via blogs, wikis, email, and face-to-face sharing, can be very valuable for disseminating a project. Today, many people can be reached through social media rather than through more traditional methods. In social networking, the message is more personal and more reflective of opinion based on evidence rather than limited to the evidence itself. In all social networking, presenters must be keenly aware of the audience, group dynamics, and spread of information.

Written reports can be very valuable means of sharing information within a system, especially if one seeks to sustain the project or innovation. This type of publication requires the author to make a more businesslike and more streamlined presentation. A business case must be made and arguments formulated to achieve sustainability. Written reports are frequently shared with internal and external audiences such as external regulators. Above all, the author of such a report should avoid verbosity and adhere to the system's guidelines.

Press releases for television, radio, and newspaper can be another valuable tool for sharing information in a more informal fashion with a more selective audience. However, if you are being interviewed in these venues rather than writing the script yourself, be aware that you may be misquoted or "bumped" if a bigger story occurs. To avoid being misquoted, make an attempt to get review privileges prior to publication; you may encounter resistance from the media outlet because timing is critical, but such a review can save you from heartache.

▶ Pitfalls in Dissemination

It is critical to be aware of two major pitfalls that can occur with any sharing of information: redundant publication and self-plagiarism. Sometimes an innovation is innovative only for one's own system and is widely accepted outside that system. Becoming an expert on the information contained in the broader literature will prevent this error.

Self-plagiarism occurs when the researcher shares the same information with more than one publication or in more than one presentation. Typically, when one is invited to present or publish, the conference or the journal becomes the owner of the information shared. Subsequent publication or presentation of the data, even if you are the researcher who discovered the findings, is problematic. Focused presentations and publications that present one finding or a very limited amount of information can prevent this faux pas and can result in multiple publications and presentations, all different, from a single study, project, or innovation.

Projects typically involve teams of contributors rather than a single researcher. Dissemination opportunities expand exponentially with the number of people involved in the project development. Sharing a common understanding of how dissemination will occur and keeping the entire team apprised of all developments is critical to limit overexposure and reduce the potential for jeopardizing the data.

Because dissemination requires an ongoing exchange of information between and among project staff, specific planning for dissemination and audiences must be addressed at the inception of project development. Several factors and conditions affecting dissemination, adoption of a project's outcome, and the sustainability of the project must be included in all presentations: the advantages that the innovation has brought to the organization; the compatibility of the innovation with the organization; the complexity of the innovation; the ability to track and observe the elements of the innovation; the inherent risks to the project; the expected reversibility and ability to revise each individual element and the project as a whole; and the leadership and support of the organization. All of these elements are based on effective communication within the organization and an assessment of the agency's readiness to change.

▶ Summary

- Dissemination of innovative projects is a natural progression of any endeavor.
- Project dissemination offers audiences new knowledge and opens up an exchange of information.
- A number of forums are available for dissemination of information, including journal publications, book chapters, and poster and podium presentations.
- Multiple presentation methods and models are available; however, the APPLE model is widely used by individuals to prepare presentations.
- Presentations using appreciative inquiry provide opportunities to share aspects of a system or project that may not be obvious to the audience.
- Careful consideration should be given to where one publishes and presents findings, who maintains the copyright, and which pitfalls of dissemination may be encountered.

Reflection Questions

1. Consider presentations you have attended in the past. What aspects engaged you? What aspects distracted you? How would you have changed the presentation had you been at the podium?
2. Which personal characteristics can impact a presentation or poster?
3. What strategies can be employed during and after a presentation to enhance the positives and decrease the negatives?
4. What actions do presenters need to take following a presentation to prepare for the next opportunity?

References

Cooperrider, D., & Whitney, D. (2010). A positive revolution in change: Appreciative inquiry. *AI Commons*. Retrieved from http://appreciativeinquiry.case.edu/intro/whatisai.cfm

Havens, D. S., Wood, S. O., & Leeman, J. (2006). Improving nursing practice and patient care: Building capacity with appreciative inquiry. *Journal of Nursing Administration, 36*(10), 463–470.

Marchionni, C., & Richer, M. C. (2007). Using appreciative inquiry to promote evidence-based practice in nursing: The glass is more than half full. *Nursing Leadership, 20*(3), 86–97.

Rutledge, P. A., Bajaj, G., & Mucciolo, T. (2007). *Special edition: Using Microsoft Office PowerPoint 2007*. Indianapolis, IN: Que.

Tappen, R. M. (2011). *Advanced nursing research: From theory to practice*. Sudbury, MA: Jones & Bartlett Learning.

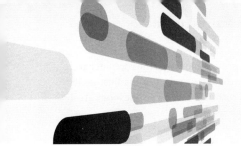

Case Exemplar

▶ Case Study 1

Presentations Supplemented with PowerPoint Tips and Examples

Catherine Dearman

PowerPoint is an instructional design tool for presentations that is commonly used, especially in business and academic settings. Because PowerPoint presentations are extensions of the traditional presentation, the typical rules for presenting evidence apply. The information that follows provides novice presenters with essential information related to PowerPoint presentations.

A PowerPoint presentation is an adjunct to the verbal presentation, and as such it needs to supplement—not replace—the presenter's oral discussion. Most instructional design specialists indicate that there should a maximum of one slide for each minute scheduled for the presentation. This basic setup includes the introductory slide, the reference slide, and the "Questions?" slide.

The basic rule of thumb for slide makeup is to include 7 lines of text with 7 words on each line (at most), for a total of 49 words per slide. At its best, the PowerPoint slide serves as a guide, prompting the presenter to mention salient points. The slides are not expected to contain every word that a presenter needs to say.

Inclusion of pictures on PowerPoint slides can be great, especially if they link to the topic at hand. For example, if the presentation is addressing community work groups building a playground, then including before, during, and after pictures would give a complete image to the audience and would replace words.

Most audiences typically prefer lighter backgrounds with darker text. Colors should complement, not detract from, the presentation.

Slide layouts sometimes intrude on the words the presenter wanted to show on the slides. Previewing the slides carefully prior to finalizing the layout will facilitate clarity and attractiveness.

Slide transitions, animation, and sound are all effective attention-getting devices. Use them cautiously, however. Not every slide needs a transition for each word. Flashing words are distracting to some viewers.

Prior to a presentation where visual aids (including PowerPoint slides) are used, the presenter is well advised to assess the environment of the presentation. Go into the room and look around. How many chairs are there? How large is the space? Is it square or rectangular? Are there impediments to full view of the screen, such as poles and projectors? Following this inspection, load the presentation onto the computer and display it. Go to the back of the room and see if the slides are clear or if adjustments in font or other elements are needed. Sometimes a color scheme for a slide looks great on a personal computer but does not communicate as well in a large group.

If the presentation is a result of funding, the funding agency typically prefers to be mentioned in some way. Some funders actually publish the statement they want used with every publication and/or presentation. Be sure to include these statements if they exist.

Index

Note: Page numbers followed by *f* or *t* indicate material in figures or tables, respectively.

A

B

C

Q